Autism: Exploring the Benefits of a Gluten- and Casein-Free Diet

Autism was once considered a rare condition, but increasing numbers of children are being diagnosed as being on the autism spectrum, making it one of the most common and often challenging childhood developmental diagnoses. While experts around the globe strive to unravel and truly understand how autism develops and presents itself, comparatively little is still known about the condition despite decades of research and investigation.

What is becoming clear is that autism is an extremely diverse condition with a presentation often complicated by a heightened risk of various accompanying behaviours and conditions outside of autism, variably affecting quality of life and future outcomes. Based on years of experimental study and thousands of personal observations, a growing body of research suggests that some challenging characteristics present in autism may be positively affected by the introduction of a gluten- and casein-free (GFCF) diet.

Autism: Exploring the Benefits of a Gluten- and Casein-Free Diet offers parents, teachers and other education or health professionals an easy-to-read alternative to sifting through the combined science. Written by leading experts in autism research, food, nutrition and dietetics, the book cuts through the jargon to offer readers a no-nonsense, accessible and authoritative overview of how diet might affect some characteristics of autism, and provides a range of useful recipes and handy hints for making mealtimes fun for children with autism and related conditions who are embarking on such a dietary change.

Paul Whiteley is a Director of ESPA Research, a subsidiary of the charity ESPA (Education and Services for People with Autism).

Mark Earnden is a chef and successful entrepreneur who is involved with several innovative food enterprises.

Elouise Robinson is a dietitian in the communit ...'' ·~ and young people.

Autism: Exploring the Benefits of a Gluten- and Casein-Free Diet

A practical guide for families and professionals

Paul Whiteley, Mark Earnden and Elouise Robinson

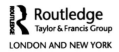
Routledge
Taylor & Francis Group

LONDON AND NEW YORK

First published 2014
by Routledge
2 Park Square, Milton Park, Abingdon, Oxon OX14 4RN

and by Routledge
711 Third Avenue, New York, NY 10017

Routledge is an imprint of the Taylor & Francis Group, an informa business

British Library Cataloguing in Publication Data
A catalogue record for this book is available from the British Library

Library of Congress Cataloging in Publication Data
Whiteley, Paul, 1972–
   Autism: exploring the benefits of a gluten- and casein-free diet : a practical guide
   for families and professionals / Paul Whiteley, Mark Earnden, Elouise Robinson.
   pages cm
   1. Autistic children—Nutrition. 2. Autism in children—Diet therapy. 3. Gluten-free diet.
   4. Casein-free diet. I. Earnden, Mark. II. Robinson, Elouise. III. Title.
   RJ506.A9W463 2014
   618.92'858820654—dc23
   2013043281

ISBN: 978–0–415–72762–4 (hbk)
ISBN: 978–0–415–72763–1 (pbk)
ISBN: 978–1–315–77791–7 (ebk)

Typeset in Bembo
by Swales & Willis Ltd, Exeter, Devon

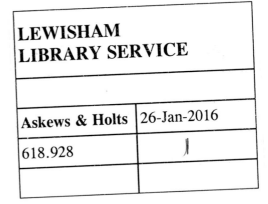

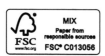

MIX
Paper from
responsible sources
FSC® C013056
www.fsc.org

Printed and bound in Great Britain by
TJ International Ltd, Padstow, Cornwall

Dedications

Elouise Robinson

To all the people in my life who love, support and inspire me, thank you. Thank you for being my initial recipe testers: your feedback has helped me shape the recipes and advice within this book.

Mark Earnden

I would like to dedicate this book to Anna, who is not only my wife but my best friend and a truly incredible person. Anna has continually been a huge source of inspiration, guidance and support throughout all my business commitments, projects and dreams. I would also like to thank my daughter Ella who has enabled me to look at my priorities in life and my family who have often inspired me and always offered their support to me over the years. I would also like to thank Louise Hardy from the Business Innovation Centre, Sunderland who introduced me to Paul, without which this book would never have been realised. Finally, I thank Percy Hedley for introducing me to a world I never knew existed, that has enriched my life for almost a decade now and was the spark behind this idea. This book is for you all.

Paul Whiteley

I would like to thank Paul Shattock OBE, friends and colleagues at ESPA (Education & Services for People with Autism), ESPA Research and the Robert Luff Foundation for giving me the opportunity and support to become a part of this book. To the many hundreds of people with autism and their families and caregivers that I've had the privilege of meeting, discussing with, and learning from over my autism research career, I offer my sincere thanks. You've shown me how rich humanity really is. To my family, Kalli, Efi, Athena and Spiros: είστε η ζωή μου.

Contents

Figures

Recipes

Introduction

Not any old science book

Don't be scared but this is a book about science

Just before you put this book down muttering the words 'I'm not a scientist' or 'I don't do science', we're going to tell you that you are a scientist and yes, you do science, even if you might not know it. Everyday you 'do' science: broadly defined as the acquisition of knowledge. It might be something as simple as deciding which route to take to work based on the traffic report evidence or testing out that new 'superfood' choice on yourself or your loved ones. We're all part-scientist. Even your very youngest children have the scientific glint in their eye as they hypothesis-test their way throughout their development and the world. Not all their experiments work by the way, but they learn and develop knowledge as a result.

But this is not any old science book. It's a science book which aims to fuse science and cookery together with a spotlight on the autism spectrum and a growing fascination with specific dietary interventions potentially impacting on the presentation of some cases of autism. Food for the mind and body you might say.

Strange, you might, think that a science book should also include some cookery. Strange too that we are talking about a condition like autism, manifesting behavioural symptoms, in relation to a cookbook. But believe it or not, diet in relation to autism has been discussed for quite a few years.

In this book, we're going to delve into the history of some of that dietary research with a specific focus on the use of a **gluten- and casein-free (GFCF) diet**; that is a diet free from **gluten** found in the cereal grains wheat, barley and rye, and **casein**, the primary protein found in various forms of animal milk. We're going to talk generally about the label of autism, how symptoms manifest and some of the relevant issues pertinent to food and eating. We're going to discuss some of the experimental studies that have been done looking at diet and autism, the mechanisms proposed to account for some of the results obtained, and how, as peculiar as it might seem, diet might be able to do so much more than influence our physical health.

> We're even going to provide some delicious recipes which are gluten- and casein-free covering various different occasions which might also be useful for others outside of any interest in autism. Science and cookery all in one place.

Indeed, outside of the science of autism and diet, the emphasis is very much on this book being a practical, interactive tool as a function of those tasty recipes you'll find dotted around the chapters and the strategies we're going to be talking about to try and make mealtimes easier and fun.

If you like our recipes we would also invite you to have a look at the website which accompanies this book: **www.thepracticalbookcompany.com** and join the club which offers more information and tasty recipes for the whole family.

If we've already given you enough confidence to proclaim that 'I do science' we'll make the related points that (a) you can cook, even if you've perhaps convinced yourself that you can't, and (b) the recipes we offer have been specially designed and chosen to be simple and affordable. So please, be brave and take back control of your cooker.

Science is . . .

To reiterate, don't be scared by the word 'science' if it conjures up images of bubbling test-tubes or science-type characters walking around laboratories in white coats talking a whole new language of science-speak. It's not all like that we promise, but there are a few principles to bear in mind.

Science is all about probability. That is measuring whether something is more or less likely to happen in a particular group of people naturally or as a consequence of a particular intervention. Science is generally not about absolutes. Always be a little bit wary when you hear the words 'scientifically proven' as if somehow promoting certainty in science, particularly when it comes to people and health.

Science is also a dynamic process with new research emerging on a daily basis. So whilst today you might hear that condition X is affected by intervention Y, don't be surprised if you come across something reporting quite different tomorrow, alongside learning about the value of replication – doing the same experiment or study more than once – and the phrase 'correlation does not equal causation'.

Science uses many tools at its disposal. This includes the use of human and animal 'subjects' depending on the branch of science, the question being asked and the technique being used. Right or wrong, there are occasions when humans cannot be used for a particular study purpose; for example, when initially testing a new medicine or where investigations involve vital organs such as the brain. Obviously animals are not humans, and animal models trying to recreate human conditions therefore represent an estimate at best.

Finally and importantly, not all science is equal. Someone shouting from the rooftops about their 'Eureka' moment that X causes or helps Y might not be the same as someone quietly publishing the results of a controlled clinical trial in a journal reviewed by their peers. There are also various degrees of scientific 'proof' ranging from the case study to the open trial all the way up to the gold standard that is the randomised, placebo-controlled, cross-over trial. Even better are two or more replications of a gold-standard trial showing similar results topped off by a meta-analysis combining all the data together. But also remember that people are not all the same . . . one man's meat is another man's poison (similarly applied to women too).

We are going to be provocative in this book about the topic of autism and the whole area of dietary intervention set within the confines of the available science. We're going to make you think about the spectrum of autism and hopefully challenge some of the dogma which has built up about the condition, its description and nature, over the years. We'll try and stay as current as we possibly can in the science we talk about in this book but readers are well advised to become their own researchers and, as time allows, keep up to date with the new science as it emerges.

We should add that we will talk about words and concepts in the book which readers might not be readily familiar with. So, if you don't know your **DNA** from your **epigenetics** or **zonulin** from *Sutterella*, we advise you to have a look at the glossary provided at the end of this book or trawl through the references to additional reading we provide or seek other sources of information on the topics in question. In addition, all the terms listed in the glossary are highlighted in **bold** in the text when they first appear in each chapter, just so you know that help is at hand if you don't happen to have a PhD in molecular biology or something related. Look to the glossary, people. We've also included some 'interesting' diagrams and summary boxes intermixed with the text in various parts of the book to try and make things more 'bite-sized'. We promise we'll try not to blind you with too much science-speak.

We don't do medical advice

So now you know what to expect from this book, here are a few words about what we are not going to do. First things first: *nothing included in this book is intended as medical or related clinical advice.* We're not medical doctors and you, our readers, are not our patients. By all means have a conversation with your medical physician about some of the concepts and ideas we talk about in this book if you wish. But please, don't start or end the conversation with the words 'but the book said I should'. If you likewise happen to be a doctor or other healthcare professional reading this book, please also note our caveat.

Next, although the GFCF diet is a primary focus of this book, we're not necessarily suggesting that the recipes we've included in it should represent the sum total of your diet for the rest of your days. We very much hope you'll enjoy making and eating the foods we present but would like to make it very clear that they are a starting point of ideas as part of a dietary regime. Oh, and sorry that we have to mention it, if you are going to attempt our recipes, please make sure that you're careful in the kitchen – your culinary laboratory. If you also have established food allergies, just double-check the ingredients we list to make sure they're safe for you.

Moving on, we're also not going to advocate that a GFCF diet is a cure-all for autism. It's not. We're not going to make sweeping claims that all autism is a dietary or any other unifying condition. It's not. We're not even going to advocate that a GFCF diet is a must-try for everyone on the autism spectrum. It's not. For all these sweeping statements, there are plenty of other books, websites, blogs, and discussion groups out there to go to. Just not here. Oh and just for the record, we're even going to resist the temptation to name the diet after ourselves. Being provocative is not the same as thinking that this book is going to be a 'game-changer' when it comes to how autism is viewed. We didn't write this book to change the world; rather to inform and make you think.

What we will advise, however, is that if you are considering making the switch to a GFCF diet or indeed making any important change to your or your family's diet, you might want to seek some medical and professional dietetic advice first. You might be questioning why you should speak to your doctor before making a dietary switch; surely it's only a change of diet? Well, you'd surprised how much of our modern diet is made up of foods which contain gluten and casein.

Despite our discussions in this book focusing on potential issues with these foodstuffs in relation to some cases of autism, they are nevertheless providers of important nutrients, **vitamins** and **minerals**. A little more knowledge about some of the alternative ways and means to ensure that such nutrients can find their way into your diet has got to be a good thing. Bear in mind also that your medical doctor might want to run a few tests before the diet is started to rule out things like **coeliac disease**, or celiac disease if you prefer the alternative spelling (we'll talk about this later on in the book).

What are gluten and casein?

Gluten is a storage protein found in various cereal grains such as wheat, barley and rye. A mixture of gliadin and glutenin, gluten is credited with helping give bread its characteristic dough-like texture. Gluten is present in various foods and drinks: breads, pasta, cakes, beers and some breakfast cereals. It can also be present in a variety of other foods working as a thickening or flavouring agent. Foods should normally be labelled according to whether they contain gluten.

Casein is a protein found in mammalian milk sources. Different variations of the casein protein are found in different animals (humans, cows, sheep, goats, etc.). Casein protein is not the same as **lactose**, which is the sugar found in milk. Casein is present in milk and other dairy products such as cheese and yoghurt.

Both gluten and casein are quite widely found in the modern diet. Various kinds of foods are naturally gluten- and casein-free including meats, fish, fruits, vegetables, various oils like olive oil and grains like rice and lentils. There is an increasingly thriving gluten-free market providing gluten-free alternatives to bread and other foods. Non-mammalian sources of milk such as rice, soya and almond milks are also commonly available alternatives.

Who do we think we are?

So who are we, why are we qualified to write this book and what makes this book different from others talking about similar things? We, the authors, are a diverse group of people: a chef, a dietitian and a researcher. We bring various skills to this book based on eating well for maintaining health and wellbeing, turning food preparation into something to be savoured rather than a chore, and interpreting science from the viewpoint of someone who has done a fair bit of science and science communication. Our common ground is translating our passion for our respective areas and making this book as enjoyable and informative as we can make it. We've all brought our skills to bear on a topic which has generated more than its fair share of discussion and controversy down the years: can diet affect cases of autism?

Before getting together to write this book, we all had a similar vision about bringing science, food and nutrition together but we each needed the others to make the dream a reality and, more importantly, credible. We knew our vision, we knew our idea was going to be innovative, and we knew the concept was much needed . . . what we didn't know was each other. We'd all like to think it was fate which brought a chef, a dietitian and an autism researcher together, but in reality it was some chance introductions which set us on a journey to write this book.

Get on with it

Obviously we'd love you to read this entire book, page for page, making it your go-to reference for anything and everything autism- and diet-related. As a general guide, the chapters making up Part I of the book are directed towards the definition of autism and stressing just how complicated a label/diagnosis/condition/disorder/disability (delete as appropriate) it really is. It might seem like we've dedicated a lot of time to the idea of 'understanding autism' but hopefully you'll see how relevant it is to the dietary story. The chapters included in Part II are focused more on the dietary side of things and where research is up to at the time of writing. Again, there is a lot of information packed into this part of the book simply because there is a lot of research out there which is relevant. Part III is the more practical part of the book. It's all about the often complicated relationship between food and autism and how small and subtle changes can often lead to easier mealtimes. We'll also be talking about the more practical aspects related to getting started with the GFCF diet should you decide the diet is for you and yours. Don't be surprised if, however, you keep reading about how we'll be coming back to particular topics in different chapters throughout the book, representative of the multitude of meeting points for various ideas and themes. Now you know a little bit of the background to this book, how about we start our journey together.

Part I

Understanding autism

Chapter 1

What is autism? (Or hello or goodbye)

Autism means different things to different people

Depending on how you view our description of autism and the autism spectrum in this opening chapter may very well influence whether you read on to the end or find alternative uses for this book very early on. Whether we use the term 'person with autism' or 'autistic person' to denote the ownership of autism, or whether we talk about 'difference' or 'disability' is likely to have some bearing on how you interpret the picture of autism we present.

Of course we're very much hoping that you will continue reading as we try to offer as broad and scientifically accurate a picture as we can of modern-day autism and our particular interest in the condition with a focus on diet and food. That being said, coupled with the often strong views held about autism and what it does and doesn't mean to someone, it is highly unlikely that we will please all of the people all of the time so again, we reiterate that autism means different things to different people.

Dr Tom Insel, at the time of writing current director of the US National Institute for Mental Health (NIMH), quite nicely summed up the issues of differing opinions and views of autism in his blogpost on '*The Four Kingdoms of Autism*'.[1] His discussions make mention of the **heterogeneity** – the wide diversity of presentation – that exists under the umbrella term 'autism' and how this diversity has lead to certain ideological divisions which fuel the different kingdoms of thought. Importantly he talks about the concept of

> Four Kingdoms of Autism (Insel, 2013)
> Illness
> Identity
> Injury
> Insight

autism as a plural condition, whereby behavioural characteristics dynamically manifest across a spectrum of ability and disability potentially due to more than one different factor in different people. Readers may do well to keep in mind the concept of 'the autisms' in subsequent chapters of this book.

To a healthcare or health-related professional engaged in diagnosing a person or researching the condition, the term autism might be taken to mean a neurodevelopmental condition including a collection of behavioural symptoms, reflecting a diagnostic dyad of impairments: communication and social interactive issues (cumulatively known as **social affect**) and the presence of restricted and repetitive behaviours (see page 10 for a summary of the core features of autism). Allied to an agreed timescale of symptom onset appearing in early infancy or childhood, autism represents a disorder of development, lies along a spectrum and is generally taken to be a lifelong label.

Some readers might question our use of the word 'dyad' to denote only two core symptoms associated with an autism diagnosis where traditionally autism was defined by a triad of symptoms. We respond to such a question by referencing the latest version of one of the primary diagnostic schedules – the Diagnostic and Statistical Manual or **DSM**[2] – and the fanfare that has greeted the arrival of DSM-5. The merging of core issues in the domains related to the use of communication and social interaction into the super domain of social affect is reflective of one of several changes made to the DSM-5 description of autism[3]. The other commonly used schedule for diagnosing autism is the **ICD (International Classification of Diseases)** criteria published by the World Health Organization (WHO). Like many other conditions currently labelled solely on the strength of a person's actions and behaviours alongside a look at historical notes and other information, diagnosing an **autism spectrum disorder (ASD)** is often part medicine, part societal and strangely enough part art.

> **Schedules for diagnosing autism**
> DSM (Diagnostic & Statistical Manual)
> ICD (International Classification of Diseases)

To a person living with autism and their family/caregivers, the term autism may reflect a slightly different description at different times across the lifespan. Depending on the severity of presented symptoms, whether the person has spoken language or capacity in other communicative skills, the likelihood of lifelong support being required and the presence or not of various comorbid conditions which can also affect quality of life, autism may carry a different meaning outside of the cold, hard diagnostic facts.

To some on the autism spectrum and their advocates, autism is to be viewed as a difference not a disability. A difference in how the world is perceived by them and indeed how they are perceived by the world around them. The focus is on accepting all kinds of minds and the neurodiversity which that entails including the message that autism is not just a condition of disorder. Building upon the disability rights movement, the emphasis is also on providing appropriate awareness and support such that autism is seen and incorporated as part of the colourful tapestry of behaviour and functioning which make up society.

In other cases, autism, its presentation and its elevated risk of comorbidities, very definitely reflects a disability. The emphasis is on how the core and other peripheral symptoms presenting in autism, sometimes in quite severe forms, can so fundamentally affect a person and their daily living. When we speak of disability, we use the term to denote that the presentation of autism so significantly impacts on a person's life that it does not allow them to fully participate in activities typical of their peers or indeed, places them at greater risk of poorer health or quality of life outcomes.

Core features of autism

Please note that this description does not serve to represent the formal diagnostic features of autism but instead describes the core features as they may present.

- *Difficulty with language and communication*
  - The development and appropriate use of verbal and non-verbal language.
  - The use of or interpretation of facial expressions or other communicative acts.
  - Difficulties understanding the nuances or conventions of social communication (e.g. turn-taking during conversation, literality of meaning).

- *Difficulty with social interaction*

  ○ Understanding and using appropriate gestures to regulate social interaction.
  ○ Issues with recognising and understanding the emotions and feelings of other across different social situations.
  ○ Difficulties with the development of peer relationships.

- *Restricted and repetitive behaviours*

  ○ Issues with engaging in appropriate play or related activities particularly with an imaginative component (instead showing a preoccupation with non-functional elements).
  ○ The presence of encompassing preoccupations which are unusually intense.
  ○ Adherences to rituals and routines which are often compulsive in nature and produce resistance and/or distress when changed.

Distinct from Dr Insel's description of separate kingdoms making up the autism landscape, the various ways that autism is described or talked about by the same person might not necessarily anchor that person to one particular viewpoint. It is fair to say that even when viewed as a disability, autism is still a cause for ensuring appropriate awareness, equality, rights and access to any services required. Likewise, the focus on autism as difference not disability does not exclude discussions on the very real day-to-day impact that the condition and/or its risk of comorbidities can have on a person. Indeed even opinions about autism are generally spectral rather than opposites, and with the rise and rise of the Internet and social media, everyone seemingly has a view.

Autism is not a failure to develop

Autism is a pervasive developmental condition. That is, the cluster of symptoms defining the condition is generally taken to appear and manifest in infancy or early childhood. From a diagnostic point of view, symptoms have to be present before the age of 3 years old, although with the arrival of the DSM-5 this very definite cut-off point has been relaxed to some degree.

It is important to understand that the symptoms of autism and the developmental focus of symptoms are not meant to imply that autism represents a complete failure to develop. Everyone develops. Whilst this might seem slightly at odds with certain characteristics such as the potential issues with failing to obtain spoken language in some cases for example, it is perhaps more relevant to suggest that autism represents a shift in developmental trajectory. Many if not all of the core symptoms present in autism are variably observed during typical development at differing times and under different situations, modified by all manner of factors. It is the intensity and persistence of such behaviours which marks them out as different in cases of autism and how their presence impacts over the course of a lifetime.

Likewise, the description of autism as being a pervasive condition highlights how fundamentally such differences in development are able to affect a person. Compared with other developmental conditions such as the speech and language disorders where problems are more restricted in scope, the wide ranging behavioural manifestations present in autism hint at its pervasive identity.

The (sometimes rocky) diagnostic path

As any parent or child developmental specialist will tell you, children are very rarely the same in the way they grow up and develop skills. Infancy and early childhood is epitomised by non-continuous patterns of new skills starting and stopping; some days a child seems to have ceased trying to better itself, other days, a whole raft of new skills seemingly come at once as parents scramble to photograph, video and document those milestones. Yes, there are general stages of development which have been defined down the years, but children don't generally follow specific timetables or concrete developmental regulations. This point serves to illustrate the difficulty in reaching one of the hallowed goals of autism research: the early behavioural identification of autism.

The (sometimes) rocky pathway towards a child being assessed and receiving a diagnosis of autism if indicated has been discussed many times over in the voluminous literature on autism. In the most part it starts with parental concerns about their child. Some parents have talked about how they knew something was 'not right' with their child from its earliest days. This includes thoughts and recollections on how their child did not seem to be reactive to the world around them, didn't seem to cry when it should have been crying or just seemed to be slightly detached. Other parents have talked about a gradual fall into autism. They describe a child who seemed to be hitting all their early milestones but as time went on didn't seem to keep up with their peers in terms of the quality of their developmental progress. Other parents report children who were progressing well, hitting all their developmental milestones and suddenly regress: losing previously acquired skills, sometimes in quite a dramatic fashion.

These examples serve to reiterate just how complex a task it is to isolate early generalisable behavioural red flags to spot potential cases of autism. For those cases where onset appears to be very early and it is clear that the 'typical' developmental trajectory is not being followed, one can see the potential for an autism 'early warning' system being in place. Indeed, as previously detailed, the focus on early social-communicative functions such as eye contact and later the various types of pointing skills, seems to be a promising area for markers of early identification of autism. For others, particularly those who present with regression as part of their symptom profile, such a system is unlikely to be of much benefit.

> **Potential red flags for autism:**
> **Social communication**
> **e.g. eye contact, pointing**

Regression!

Ah yes, regression. Not only the potential fly in the ointment for those developmental red flag 'here comes autism' systems but a part of the autism spectrum which has certainly seen its fair share of discussion and controversy down the years.

It's fair to say that the recognition of regression – a loss of previously acquired skills – when it comes to the onset of autism, has not had the easiest of times. Regression as part of conditions like Heller's syndrome otherwise known as **childhood disintegrative disorder (CDD)** has been known about for over a hundred years. Indeed, if readers are so minded, we can very much recommend reading the translation and interpretation of Theo Heller's original 1908 paper by Westphal and colleagues[4] and see how close Heller actually came to describing autism (over 30 years before Kanner).

Regression in the early days of autism was talked about, just not necessarily with the presentation of autism centrally in mind. So, early papers described regression due to **epilepsy** or regression due to other conditions like Rett syndrome. Around about the 1990s behavioural regression accompanying a diagnosis of autism started to get a little more research attention alongside the realisation that regression wasn't just some rare occurrence as was once thought. Some of the latest estimates for regression, bearing in mind regression can cover lots of different skills, suggest that about a quarter to a third of children with autism seem to experience some kind of loss of skills[5] coincidental to the onset of symptoms.

Regression in relation to autism onset can take many forms. Language skills, social skills (acknowledging that the DSM-5 social affect category bundles these areas together) and other, more non-core symptoms have all been reported to be affected by regression. Research has even reported a mixed model of delays + regression as seemingly apparent for some children.[6]

The reports of regression in cases of autism also ask some interesting questions about the aetiology and nature of autism for some people. One could assume that regression might be pre-programmed for some children, where, alongside other variables such as head size[7] which has also been talked about with autism in mind, there may be subtle genetic or **epigenetic** triggers which set forth a gradual sequence of events characterised by regression resulting in autism. One might also assume that regression may be representative of something rather more environmentally weighted such as the effects of infection or other pathogenic insult. The model here following something similar to the description of PANDAS (pediatric autoimmune neuropsychiatric disorders associated with streptococcal infections)[8] or **PANS (pediatric acute-onset neuropsychiatric syndrome)** where for example, childhood-onset **obsessive–compulsive disorder (OCD)** has been linked to Group A beta-haemolytic streptococcal infections. That being said, the precise type of pathogen (bacterial, viral or toxicological) is still a source of some discussion and debate. One might even speculate that other environmental changes during the early years such as a change towards a more adult-style diet might also be involved (or not)?

What causes autism? Insert idea here: _____

The question of how autism comes about has similarly created kingdoms of differing opinions. To again use the term the 'autisms', the implication is that behind the common bond of the dyad of behavioural manifestations, the experience of autism is not the same for everyone. The heterogeneity or diversity of presentation, which itself is dynamic throughout the lifespan, perhaps signal that universal factors of 'causation' based on our current categorisation of autism are going to be limited.

The older psychological theories of autism being due to refrigerator parenting styles or other psychoanalytical interpretations have, in the most part, been consigned to the annals of history. The current view is that autism comes about as a consequence of

> Autism comes about as a consequence of the variable interplay between genes and environment

an interplay between genetic and environmental factors.[9] Such interplay being variable in weighting across different people according to factors, such as any family history of autism or related conditions or the potential risks from various implicated external events.

As with many things related to autism, the precise details of these internal and external factors of causation are still the source of some speculation. The problems of defining autism based on checklists of characteristics have done little to aid in teasing out aetiological factors. So for example, there is no single gene or genetic mutation associated with all cases of autism,[10] just as no single environmental factor is acting on the developing baby or during the early years of all children destined to be diagnosed with autism. There are however promising lines of scientific investigation emerging from the mountains of research being done on what might cause autism.

Genetics and epigenetics

Figure 1.1 provides a brief overview of the science of genetics. Humans like other organisms are designed and produced to a blueprint or genetic map. The code of that blueprint is **DNA** – deoxyribonucleic acid. DNA is present in nearly every cell of the body and is made up of a code consisting of four core chemicals: adenine (A), guanine (G), cytosine (C) and thymine (T), forming rungs of the DNA ladder. Your DNA is inherited from both your parents and determines lots of different features which make you individual, such as eye and hair colour.

Your DNA is generally unique to you except if you have an identical twin. When someone talks about a condition being genetic, it normally implies that there is some problem with the DNA blueprint which, because DNA controls the production of important chemicals in the body, either interferes with typical body functions or places that person at greater risk of certain conditions or diseases.

The current scientific consensus is that autism most likely includes a genetic component in its aetiology. We say this not to apportion blame or to make any sweeping gener-

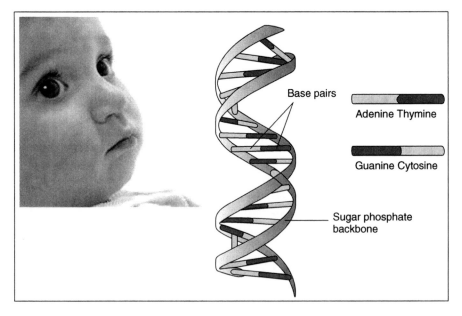

Figure 1.1 DNA: the genetic code.

alisations that autism is a wholly genetic condition in the same way that Down syndrome or **Fragile X syndrome** is. But the evidence does point to some kind of genetic effect potentially being involved, despite the fact that the details of which genes show involvement and the mode of heredity are still a little sketchy.

We're conscious that this last statement might sound a little anti-science. We say science knows that 'autism has a genetic component' but in the same breath say it does not know what it is and has yet to provide totally convincing evidence of its effect. Talk about a faith in science eventually coming up with the goods. To clarify, some of the reasons why science has come to the conclusion that autism might have some genetic roots have relied upon studies of identical (monozygotic) and non-identical (dizygotic) twins[11] for example and the concordance rates of one or both twins presenting with autism. The fact that, in addition, various genetic glitches, i.e. small changes in the genetic code, have been reported in relation to cases of autism[12] also reflects the involvement of genes, together with the presentation of autistic-like behaviours in genetic conditions like Fragile X syndrome and indeed more recently discovered genetic conditions, some of which we'll talk about later. The idea of a broader **phenotype** of autism (more also on that later) adds further weight to some involvement for the building blocks of life being involved. The funding priorities for autism research have, as a result, been very heavily skewed in favour of genetic research.

It could be argued, however, that those who suggest autism is a wholly genetic condition are perhaps oversimplifying what is an extremely complex area. Aside from the issues of heterogeneity and **comorbidity**, which you'll be hearing more about in the coming chapters, recent research looking at the rates of autism in twins has to some degree revised the argument that twins from one egg are both absolutely 100 per cent predestined to develop autism as a function of their identical genomes if the autism-related genes, whatever they are, are present.[13] The idea that autism is wholly genetic also flies in the face of the increasing numbers of cases of autism being reported, assuming that some kind of traditional Mendelian inheritance pattern might pertain. Further discussion about this topic follows.

Outside of the idea that humans do not walk around with all their genes permanently switched to the on or off position, the science of genetics is continually making some advances in knowledge about our genome and how it works. The relatively recent introduction of the science of **epigenetics**, starting in earnest within the past decade, is testament to the fact that the genome we are born with might not just on its own be a blueprint for our future health and risk of disease or ill-health.[14] Whilst there is still some confusion about what constitutes the epigenome and the science of epigenetics, an oft-cited phrase is that your genes might not necessarily be your destiny. The idea is that over and above that genetic instruction manual inherited from your parents, there exists a series of modifying chemicals which have the ability to influence the activation or not of certain genes. Several processes fit this epigenetic bill including gene **methylation** and related actions and histone modification – that is, altering the chemicals which keep DNA neatly packaged up so able to fit into the minute space which is a cell nucleus.[15]

> Epigenetics refers to the ways that expression of your genes can be chemically modified

Already in these very early days of the epigenetic study of autism, scientific interest is growing. The available results emerging also point to several important potential effects related for example, to methylation patterns as a whole[16] and also with regards to specific genes in specific organs of the body. At the same time, **epigenetic** findings should be viewed as complementary to the more traditional structural genomic changes that have already been reported in cases of autism. We'll also perhaps introduce you to the concepts of the 'jumping genes' and genomic hotspots at this point and their relationship to our viral forefathers – **HERVs (human endogenous retroviruses)** – without venturing too far into these areas in this book.

Whilst it is difficult to conclude at the present time exactly where the involvement of the genome and epigenome might be heading with autism in mind, what is clear is that their contribution is likely very complex. If one is to assume that gene expression can be chemically modified or that mutations in genes found in cases of autism but not their parents – described as *de novo* – might not just be a random spontaneous action but occurring as part of the ageing process of parents for example, one then also corroborates the idea that genes might not work alone but rather in unison with more environmental factors too.

Environment

Like genetics, environment is a nebulous term. To say that the beginnings of a condition like autism might come about as a result of environmental factors opens the door to a multitude of possible issues being involved. It is generally implied that the meaning of environment focuses on some external force or forces acting singly or cumulatively upon the risk of a person developing autism or other condition. This however means that anything and everything which is not innate, naturally included in our cells during our earliest days, is up for grabs as potentially being related.

One can perhaps see how such a wide-ranging term adds an even more significant degree of complexity to the question of autism causation. To say environment is contributory to autism also leaves the door open to sometimes strange ideas being discussed, as was the case with those previous psychogenic schools of thought. Generally, however, modern interpretations of environmental factors influencing autism risk have settled on key areas and stages of interest: our earliest days *in utero*, our 'chemical' romance and various facets of the physical world around us.

Despite the tremendous medical advances being made to keep our children safe whilst inside the watery cocoon during the nine months that makes them, the developing foetus is still a fragile entity. Solely dependent on their mothers for nourishment and protection, the developing child is vulnerable at every stage of pregnancy and parturition (birth) to infections, physical trauma and exposure events of many different kinds. As shown by the examples of foetal alcohol syndrome (FAS), neural tube defects and the very unfortunate thalidomide episode, what mum is exposed to can sometimes have a devastating effect on foetal development.

Baby, baby

Needless to say that various foetal exposure events have been correlated with the elevated risk of offspring developing autism. Viral insults such as rubella represent the more classic association[17] with cases of autism but other infections are also thought to increase risk too.[18] Without getting too caught up on individual viruses or bacteria as being potential risk factors, quite of a lot of focus has shifted to the processes of how maternal immune activation, possibly as a result of such infections, might impact on whether offspring will subsequently be diagnosed with autism. Paul Patterson and his team have been particularly active in this growing area of research interest[19] (more on him later).

Chemical reaction

The word 'chemical' in relation to environmental factors potentially modifying the risk of autism has, perhaps, more than any other word been misunderstood. Everything that we are and everything around us is some form of chemical. The food we eat, the water we drink, the medicines we take all comprise of chemicals. Chemicals were life yesteryear and chemicals are life today. The mix-up has primarily occurred because of the way the word chemical has been used to infer something 'synthetic and unnatural' as opposed to something 'green and natural', even though strictly speaking, both are of the same family.

That's not to say however that there aren't a wide range of chemicals in the form of medicines and other chemical classes which might have the propensity to modify the risk of autism. The various investigations being done on the use of pre- and peri-conceptual use of **folic acid** represents one such example. Pregnant mums will no doubt have heard about how folic acid supplementation reduces the risk of neural tube defects (such as spina bifida) in the developing foetus and been asked to supplement with **vitamin** B9 (folic acid). There is now growing evidence that folic acid may also offset the risk of autism[20] particularly it seems, where specific genetic issues might already exist (see our later discussion on something called **MTHFR**).

Similarly, the role of various medicines specifically when taken during pregnancy has come under the research spotlight where risk of autism is concerned. Valproate or valproic acid, a medicine normally used to control epilepsy, is one such example, with the suggestion that its use under certain circumstances may elevate the risk of offspring autism.[21] Although the specific mode of action associated with greater risk of offspring autism is still under investigation, it may be potentially relevant to note that valproate has some epigenetic actions outside of just reducing seizure activity. Please note that we do not advocate changing any patterns of prescription drugs on the basis of your reading such information here. Speak to your supervising physician if you are worried and, importantly, don't mess around with the management of epilepsy. There are a myriad of other chemicals and chemical breakdown products, some readily classed as pollutants, which have also been correlated to autism risk[22] all requiring more comprehensive study including any synergistic effects.

Pollution and residues

Various other facets of the environment have also been investigated with a view to autism risk. Air pollution and, in particular, maternal proximity to air pollution such as small particulate matter during pregnancy, is emerging as a potentially important environmental factor.[23] Often met by a rolling of the eyes and the words 'we're all exposed to air pollution', the statistical correlations being reported based on various database information are however a worthy candidate for more detailed study.

Another focus for research linking environmental factors to elevated autism risk is that of residues and metabolites from medicines. With ever increasing population numbers and more people taking medicines to manage a wide range of acute and chronic health conditions, it is inevitable that breakdown products from these drugs will find their way into the environment. Ever thought what happens to your pee after taking a painkiller? As such, there have been preliminary suggestions that levels of certain medicine residues may, through finding their way into our food and drinking sources, potentially affect developmental outcomes to include autism at least based on animal models.[24]

And then there are the often heated discussions on whether or not certain preventative medicines delivered in a needle during early infancy might also impact on autism risk. The epidemiological and other evidence very strongly say no.[25] A quite vocal group continue, though, to ask that inquiry into such an association not be halted for every single case of autism.[26]

What should be evident from our very concise overviews of the genetic and environmental schools of thought on autism causation is that simple assertions that autism is either one or the other are unhelpful. Indeed, the focus of the debate has for most people, shifted to how we decide the relative weighting of these titans across different people often under different circumstances. The increased focus on sub-groups or **phenotypes** within the autism spectrum – examining smaller groups of people with autism who share common features – is a very useful development when it comes to the question of what might cause autism.[27] Coupled also with the increased use of 'big data' where genetic, biochemical and other data from the –omics (sorry about the technical talk) are processed together, autism research is starting to advance towards less fuzzy ideas about how the condition might come about. But the questions of aetiology and its mechanisms have not been fully answered yet.

How many people have autism?

Allied to the discussions on what might cause autism are the equally vigorous debates on just how many people have autism and whether this number is truly increasing. The latest estimates hint that anywhere between 1 in 50 children[28] and 1 in 88 children[29] may present with an autism spectrum disorder. In some cases, the prevalence has been estimated to be even more frequent.[30] We don't think many people would argue with the fact that compared to the time of the earliest description of autism back in the 1940s[31] (or even earlier[32]) when autism was considered rare, many more people are diagnosed with autism in modern times.

There are various reasons why this is the case: the diagnostic criteria that are used to identify autism and how wide a diagnostic net they cast, the increasing awareness of autism and how modern trends in diagnosis have reclassified people who once would have been diagnosed with a learning disability or other condition as now having an autism label. The issue of whether there has been a real increase in cases outside of these factors is where the arguments persist.[33] Linked also to the debate on how much of autism is genes and how much is environment, any suggestions of a real increase in cases could conceivably shift the balance of causation further away from a purely genetic answer.

Included in the debate on how many people have autism is the question of differences in the rates of autism as a function of factors such as gender and geography. Perhaps the most commonly cited statistic about autism is the seemingly quite startling difference when it comes to how many more boys are diagnosed with autism compared with girls. A ratio of 4:1 boys:girls is often reported although even this figure is disputed.[34] Such a disparity could indicate some difference in the risk of autism between the sexes, and indeed various investigations have included this variable as part of their analysis (e.g. the chromosomal differences between men and women).

> More boys than girls are diagnosed with autism (4:1 ratio)

But, as so often happens in autism research, things might not necessarily be all that they seem. Questions, for example, have arisen about whether the sex differences in diagnosis rates have fully taken into consideration differences in the behavioural presentation of autism in girls and boys. Or indeed, whether being female might confer some level of protection against developing autism rather than the risk just being higher for boys. Likewise the question of differing rates of autism among different groups of people based on geography and ethnicity has also been debated. In particular, whether migration might play a modifying role in autism risk.[35] All of this set against the background of those 'autisms'.

You get the message

After reading this first chapter you should probably be getting a flavour for how complicated things are when it comes to talking about autism and the autism spectrum. We've talked about how autism means different things to different people but not necessarily being a static opinion, how we still know very little about what might cause autism, and how even a fairly straightforward question like 'how many people have autism' is fraught with differences and debate. In the next chapter, we're going to talk about the issues of individuality and comorbidity with autism in mind. We'll also discuss the various ways and means that science has been trying to intervene to improve quality of life for those on the autism spectrum taking into account that diversity.

But not so fast. Just before you head over to the next chapter, you'll note that we end each chapter with a list of references covering some of the topics discussed. It's all part of the science: providing readers with something to substantiate our arguments and give you an opportunity to do some further reading and if necessary, disagree with us. In fact, the reference list is an essential part of science, particularly those references from the peer-reviewed scientific literature; many of which can be accessed via resources such as the United States National Library of Medicine (NLM) service, PubMed. If you're not using it already, we'd encourage you to have a look: http://www.ncbi.nlm.nih.gov/pubmed

Oh, and if you're familiar with the concept of open-access publishing, we're going to try and use as many open-access references as we can so that you can read whole articles and not just the abstract. And finally... *et al.* just in case you didn't know, means 'and others' thus saving us having to list every single author on each research paper we reference.

References

1. Insel T. Blog post: *The Four Kingdoms of Autism*. National Institute of Mental Health. 2013. http://www.nimh.nih.gov/about/director/2013/the-four-kingdoms-of-autism.shtml
2. American Psychiatric Association. *Diagnostic and Statistical Manual of Mental Disorders V (DSM-V)*. Washington DC: American Psychiatric Association. 2013.
3. Volkmar F. & Reichow B. Autism in DSM-5: progress and challenges. *Molecular Autism* 2013; 4: 13.

4. Westphal A. *et al.* Revisiting regression in autism: Heller's dementia infantilis. Includes a translation of Über Dementia Infantilis. *J Autism Dev Disord.* 2013; 43: 265–271.

5. Barger BD. *et al.* Prevalence and onset of regression within autism spectrum disorders: a meta-analytic review. *J Autism Dev Disord.* 2013; 43: 817–828.

6. Ozonoff S. *et al.* Parental report of the early development of children with regressive autism: the delays-plus-regression phenotype. *Autism.* 2005; 9: 461–486.

7. Nordahl CW. *et al.* Brain enlargement is associated with regression in preschool-age boys with autism spectrum disorders. *Proc Natl Acad Sci USA.* 2011; 108: 20195–20200.

8. Swedo S. *et al.* The PANDAS subgroup: recognition and treatment. *CNS Spectr.* 2001; 6: 419–422, 425–426.

9. Chaste P. & Leboyer M. Autism risk factors: genes, environment, and gene-environment interactions. *Dialogues Clin Neurosci.* 2012; 14: 281–292.

10. Anney R. *et al.* Individual common variants exert weak effects on the risk for autism spectrum disorders. *Hum Mol Genet.* 2012; 21: 4781–4792.

11. Folstein S. & Rutter M. Infantile autism: a genetic study of 21 twin pairs. *J Child Psychol Psychiatry.* 1977; 18: 297–321.

12. Klei L. *et al.* Common genetic variants, acting additively, are a major source of risk for autism. *Mol Autism.* 2012; 3: 9.

13. Hallmayer J. *et al.* Genetic heritability and shared environmental factors among twin pairs with autism. *Arch Gen Psychiatry.* 2011; 68: 1095–1102.

14. Dodou K. & Whiteley P. DNA not necessarily your destiny? The growing role of epigenetics in pharmacy. *Pharmaceutical J.* 2013. 290: 23.

15. Annunziato AT. DNA packaging: nucleosomes and chromatin. *Nature Education.* 2008. Available at: http://www.nature.com/scitable/

16. Wong CC. *et al.* Methylomic analysis of monozygotic twins discordant for autism spectrum disorder and related behavioural traits. *Mol Psychiatry.* 2013: doi: 10.1038/mp.2013.41.

17. Chess S. Follow-up report on autism in congenital rubella. *J Autism Child Schizophr.* 1977; 7: 69–81.

18. Sweeten TL. *et al.* Brief report: autistic disorder in three children with cytomegalovirus infection. *J Autism Dev Disord.* 2004; 34: 583–586.

19. Patterson PH. Maternal infection and immune involvement in autism. *Trends Mol Med.* 2011; 17: 389–394.

20. Surén P. *et al.* Association between maternal use of folic acid supplements and risk of autism spectrum disorders in children. *JAMA.* 2013; 309: 570–577.

21. Christensen J. *et al.* Prenatal valproate exposure and risk of autism spectrum disorders and childhood autism. *JAMA.* 2013; 309: 1696–1703.

22. Landrigan P. *et al.* A research strategy to discover the environmental causes of autism and neurodevelopmental disabilities. *Environ Health Perspect.* 2012; 120: a258–a260.

23. Becerra TA. *et al.* Ambient air pollution and autism in Los Angeles county, California. *Environ Health Perspect.* 2013; 121: 380–386.

24. Thomas MA. & Klaper RD. Psychoactive pharmaceuticals induce fish gene expression profiles associated with human idiopathic autism. *PLoS One.* 2012; 7: e32917.

25. Hornig M. *et al.* Lack of association between measles virus vaccine and autism with enteropathy: a case-control study. *PLoS One.* 2008; 3: e3140.

26. Singh VK. *et al.* Abnormal measles-mumps-rubella antibodies and CNS autoimmunity in children with autism. *J Biomed Sci.* 2002; 9: 359–364.

27. Geschwind DH. Advances in autism. *Annu Rev Med.* 2009; 60: 367–380.

28. Blumberg SJ. *et al.* Changes in prevalence of parent-reported autism spectrum disorder in school-aged U.S. children: 2007 to 2011–2012. *National Health Statistics Reports.* 2013: 65.

29. Autism and Developmental Disabilities Monitoring Network Surveillance Year 2008 Principal Investigators; Centers for Disease Control and Prevention. Prevalence of autism spectrum

disorders – Autism and Developmental Disabilities Monitoring Network, 14 sites, United States, 2008. *MMWR Surveill Summ.* 2012; 61: 1–19.

30. Kim YS. *et al.* Prevalence of autism spectrum disorders in a total population sample. *Am J Psychiatry.* 2011; 168: 904–912.
31. Kanner L. Autistic disturbances of affective contact. *Nerv Child.* 1943; 2: 217–250.
32. Fitzgerald M. *Asperger's disorder.* 2008. Informa Healthcare.
33. Weintraub K. The prevalence puzzle: autism counts. *Nature.* 2011; 479: 22–24.
34. Whiteley P. *et al.* Gender ratios in autism, Asperger syndrome and autism spectrum disorder. *Autism Insights.* 2010; 2: 17–24.
35. Barnevik-Olsson M. *et al.* Prevalence of autism in children of Somali origin living in Stockholm: brief report of an at-risk population. *Dev Med Child Neurol.* 2010; 52: 1167–1168.

Chapter 2

If you've met one person with autism, you've met one person with autism

You're still here? Good. If this book is your introduction to autism – what science thinks it is and how it manifests – as well as the specific topic of dietary intervention and autism, you're probably starting to realise that when we talk about autism or the 'autisms' we are talking about quite a fuzzy concept. Part of that fuzziness stems from the diverse presentation of the condition. How for example, the autism spectrum includes people who are verbal and able to traverse the world seemingly quite independently (the emphasis being on the word 'seemingly'), and those who are almost completely reliant on others to tend to their daily living requirements. You might also appreciate how such differing presentations might be a source of those kingdom differences that we talked about in the previous chapter.

With such diversity in mind, it's little wonder that autism has been likened to things like snowflakes and clouds to convey the individuality that accompanies the condition: the focus being on the so-called N = 1 where N is the number of people and 1 is self explanatory. One of the more commonly used phrases which have tried to encapsulate this **heterogeneity** is: *If you've met one person with autism, you've met one person with autism.* Outside of just differences in the presentation of symptoms, that phrase also hints at another issue about autism with regards to how autism overlays on to a person and the question: is autism central to a person or just something comorbid?

Given the remit of this book, we have neither the space nor any great desire to go too far into this debate and the philosophical implications of each viewpoint. Once again, your perspective of the centrality of autism is to a large extent going to be influenced by your kingdom opinion. There is some movement in scientific circles starting to view autism as part of a wider series of presentations in childhood rather than just a stand-alone condition in view of the seemingly elevated risk of other developmental and indeed more somatic based conditions being present alongside autism.

The concept of the **broader autism phenotype**[36] **(BAP)** which we introduced earlier may also be relevant. The BAP denotes how that spectral view of autism and its characteristics extends outside of the diagnostic borderlands into what some might call

> The broader autism phenotype (BAP) describes less severe symptoms of autism

'normal functioning'. Obviously 'normal' is more often a point of view rather than something concrete, but again this is not a philosophical argument we want to get into with this book.

The ESSENCE of comorbidity

ESSENCE – **early symptomatic syndromes eliciting neurodevelopmental clinical examinations** – is a relatively new term being promulgated by some autism research groups.[37] The suggestion is that more often than not, when a child or even adult presents for a clinical assessment, the signs and symptoms of autism, if present, generally do not appear alone according to the prescribed diagnostic criteria. While to many this might seem like common sense – assessment for autism can be quite a complicated process – the scientific realisation that issues in relation to attention, activity levels, mood and sleep can also be present alongside the more traditional characteristics of autism is an important point.

A diagnosis of autism or autism spectrum disorder is seemingly protective of nothing. It has long been recognised that receipt of a diagnosis does seem to place a person at increased risk of developing certain other conditions. **Epilepsy** or seizure-type disorders are perhaps one of the more well-known associations that have been made.[38] Indeed, this is one of the more worrying conditions, given its very serious potential to impact on health and in some cases mortality. Features or a diagnosis of **attention deficit (hyperactivity) disorder (AD(H)D)** can also present in cases of autism,[39] as can various other developmental conditions too numerous to name here.

The concept of multiple overlapping conditions which include autism, whilst nothing new, is starting to feature more heavily in research practice too. As discussed previously, the search for the 'autism gene' has all but been put out to pasture. The simplistic notion that everyone included on the very fuzzy autism spectrum is somehow genetically united by one 'glitch' is beginning to sound very dated indeed. Research findings from other similar tick box defined conditions, ranging from ADHD to **schizophrenia**, have met with an equivalent degree of non-success when it comes to universal genetic or biological findings. It is therefore not surprising that research is moving towards not just looking at a range of genetic and environmental factors as variably impacting on different people diagnosed with autism, but also the idea that there maybe shared commonalities across different behavioural and psychiatric labels.

The possibility of common genetic ground across conditions such as autism, ADHD, schizophrenia and depression has been explored.[40] The idea of shared genetic effects which might manifest as autism in one person and schizophrenia in another or even both conditions in the same person, offers quite a radical alternative to the contemporary view. The implication is that the current system of labelling discrete conditions based on prescribed observable criteria, whilst useful for denoting difference, does very little to aid in the hunt for underlying genetics or biochemistry. Indeed, that our continued reliance on such diagnostic categorisations as research starting points almost dooms to failure any hope for a more objective, biologically based tool for identifying such difference and onwards pathogenic mechanisms. It is perhaps then not surprising that those working in autism and other areas of psychiatric research are starting to think about moves away from diagnosis as a primary variable when it comes to investigations in line with the example of **RDoC (research domain criteria)**.[41]

Schizophrenia

Having made mention of the diagnosis of schizophrenia as potentially showing some genetic overlap with autism and other conditions, it is worth passing comment on the history of the condition, with autism in mind. Variously described and defined in modern culture, schizophrenia is a chronic mental health condition which is most often diagnosed in the adolescent and early-mid adult years. The primary symptoms of schizophrenia involve the way a person perceives the reality around them. People with schizophrenia can experience hallucinations and delusions reflecting their perception of things and beliefs which are not based in reality which can alter their behaviour, corresponding to the presence of positive and negative symptoms.

> Schizophrenia is a condition which affects the way a person perceives reality

Similar to autism and various other conditions currently defined and diagnosed solely on the basis of observable symptoms and developmental history, there is no consensus on what causes schizophrenia outside of being some variable combination of genetics and environment. As exemplified by the often inaccurate representations of the condition – being 'a split mind' and the exaggerated link between violence and schizophrenia – there is still some degree of stigma attached to receiving a diagnosis of the condition despite efforts to combat the prejudice that this can bring. Combined with the way symptoms can present, and side-effects associated with some of the ways the condition is treated using particular kinds of medicines, the emerging scientific evidence suggests that people with a diagnosis of schizophrenia are at significantly greater risk of poorer social and health outcomes and an earlier death than the general population.

At one time, autism and schizophrenia were very close from a diagnostic point of view. Prior to the modern formalisation of autism as a specific diagnostic entity, it was not uncommon to hear about the label childhood schizophrenia as also describing cases which included the presentation of autism. As issues associated with the over-generalisation of the term childhood schizophrenia were more frequently discussed in scientific circles[42] so the fashion turned to separate the two diagnoses.

In more recent times, several investigators have started to closely examine the links between autism and schizophrenia and ascertain whether moves towards a complete separation of the two conditions may have been premature. Some quite startling data have emerged suggesting that, in particular groups, up to 60 per cent of people with schizophrenia may also present with symptoms which would place them on the autism spectrum.[43] Similarly, other evidence suggests that the spectrum of presentation of schizophrenia might to some degree coincide with the autism spectrum.[44] Immediately these suggestions impact on the issue of autism prevalence and in particular, the arguments for diagnostic reclassification as being part and parcel of any increase in total cases.

Acknowledging again that being placed on the autism diagnostic spectrum does not seem to be protective of any other condition developing, including those symptoms pertinent to schizophrenia such as psychosis,[45] there is a growing body of evidence showing cross-over between the range of presentation in autism and schizophrenia. Whilst such a reunion may yet impact on things like the autism-awareness message and how autism is perceived by the wider society, it does fit neatly into the proposals for common ground over and above a more fragmented general view of behaviour and psychiatry. It might also imply that outside of shared genetic features across these and other conditions, other factors may also unite the conditions or at least certain parts of the spectrums of these conditions. Interestingly, this may also include a role for food and diet and the groundbreaking work of the late Curtis Dohan (senior), which we'll be discussing in later chapters.

ADHD

Characterised by patterns of behaviour demonstrating issues with attention, activity levels and impulsiveness, **ADHD** represents probably the most prevalent childhood developmental disorder diagnosed in modern times. Estimated to affect approximately 7 per cent of children and young adults,[46] the condition, which has again been subjected to stereotyping and ridicule in some quarters of society, can significantly impact on a person's life and have potentially far-reaching consequences into adulthood.

Following a similar pattern of knowing but not-knowing about the possible causes of ADHD (yes, genes and environment variably acting in unison again), there is a growing body of research indicating that early life factors such as various exposures during pregnancy (lead, smoking, alcohol, drugs of abuse) and being born premature can adversely affect the risk of developing the condition.[47] Advice to manage or curb the more disruptive symptoms of ADHD has generally included the use of certain types of medicines alongside behavioural and other psychological interventions, although there is no current cure. As suggested previously, there is an increasing realisation that ADHD either as symptom clusters or as a diagnosis can, and does, quite frequently occur alongside cases of autism. Best estimates

> ADHD is a condition characterised by problems with attention and activity levels

have put a figure of anything up to 50 per cent of children with autism also meeting the diagnostic criteria for ADHD too.[48]

Following again a seemingly common theme, as in connection with the suggestions made in schizophrenia, there is a body of scientific work which has indicated that at least some cases of ADHD might have a link with diet and the consumption of certain foodstuffs (e.g. the **Feingold diet).** This will be discussed in more detail in subsequent chapters.

We've got to mention the brain and psychology

Quite a few of these add-on symptoms or comorbid diagnoses also substantiate why many autism research resources have been dedicated to looking at the brain as being a central organ to account for the behavioural presentation of autism. That grey-pink matter floating in our skull is a remarkable piece of bioengineering. As technology has progressed, science has been allowed greater access into the inner workings of the brain and how its electrical, biochemical, structural and genetic operations correlate with our behaviour and experiences. There is also the promise of bigger things ahead for neuroscience.[49] That all being said, research into the brain is still very much in its infancy with regards to autism, as it is with many other areas of investigation. Hindered by all that heterogeneity present in autism including conditions like epilepsy and seizure-type disorders, but also the prospect that autism might not necessarily be an exclusively brain-based condition but something rather more systemic, several alternative lines of investigation have been opened in autism research.

One cannot however talk about the brain and autism without touching upon the input that psychology has had on how autism is thought about. Psychology, or more specifically psychiatry, originally defined autism[31] and its influence has spread across the decades ever since. As mentioned, branches of psychology have also provided some of the darkest hours for autism, for instance in the writings of people such as Bruno Bettelheim and their 'blame the parents' sentiments[50] all wrapped up in the psychoanalytical blanket of thought of the time.

By comparison, more contemporary psychological theories attempting to understand the core features of autism have tended to focus more on the cognitive and behavioural features of the condition. Their attempts, utilising models drawn from developmental and cognitive psychology, were initially received with much acclaim. In more recent years, their usefulness and applicability have waned, to a large extent due to those issues with the heterogeneity of autism.[51] Also, as part of a larger reorganisation of psychology moving away from grand sweeping generalised theories about conditions like autism, psychology has lurched nearer and nearer to neuroscience and its focus on specific areas of physical and biochemical functioning over and above merely hypothetical models of conditions and diagnoses.

If any one psychological theory of autism has pre-dominated over the years, it is surely that of the **theory of mind (ToM) deficit model**.[52] Based on the assumption that autism reflects an inability or problem with understanding the intentions and beliefs of others – putting yourself into the shoes of another – ToM issues seemingly correlated well with autism, mapping on to issues with perspective taking and empathy. ToM in relation to autism continues to attract support in some quarters. Corresponding to the move towards a greater biological focus within elements of psychological science, ToM has likewise adapted. Incorporation of the involvement of the sex hormone, testosterone as accounting for the bigger ToM picture in autism has led to the suggestion of a specific cognitive style, increased systemising, with a corresponding reduction in empathetic abilities to again map on to the characteristics of autism. Indeed, several screening and assessment instruments rely on such descriptions as potentially indicating the presence of autism. Coupled with strategies to teach ToM skills, this theory is far from finished.

> A lack of theory of mind (ToM) has been suggested to be a core issue in autism

However, like much of the psychological literature and its attempts to define autism, such theories are being less and less seen as offering answers about autism. An increasingly vocal opposition to a total ToM deficit in autism, all autism, has been witnessed in recent years. It appears that notions of people with autism as being cold automatons with little or no emotion or capability to understand emotion are, to quite a large extent, wrong. Various studies have similarly hinted that universal issues with ToM in autism pay little attention to the specificity of the findings, as in issues with ToM being present in several other conditions, or indeed to the differences across different peoples and different cultures. In short and without trying to cause any offence, psychology is seemingly losing its grip on defining the essential nature of autism.

To intervene or not intervene: that is the question

Having introduced the concepts of autism as being a fairly nebulous description with cases potentially also carrying various elevated risk of **comorbidity**, we should talk a little bit about the issue of intervention and how these factors have affected the guidance on intervention. We're not specifically going to talk about dietary intervention at this point in time but rather we introduce some discussion about the concept of intervention and examples of the more 'mainstream' interventions which have been proposed and used for autism.

At the risk of overdoing the discussions about the kingdoms of autism views and opinions, one could envisage that not everyone with a connection to autism would feel particularly enamoured of the concept of intervention. Intervention implies something therapeutic. It implies that something is 'broken' and needs adjusting and/or fixing. Nowadays, most people are likely to hear the word intervention with reference to something like surgical intervention or military intervention. Both terms paint a rather intrusive picture of the concept. Indeed, for some, particularly those who might look to autism as difference not disorder, intervention is probably not going to be a cause to be celebrated.

That being said, one could, however, argue that we are intervening all the time into autism whether we realise it or not. It might be something as subtle as the way parents and teachers change their interaction style with children with autism, or the provision of social occasions and events for children and adults on the spectrum to help relieve problems of social isolation. Even the increased use of the Internet and mobile and tablet computer technologies which we are all witnessing are overlapping with the growing research base of assisted technology[53] to provide some novel solutions to issues associated with autism. Intervention is readily happening whether we see it as intervention or not.

The autism intervention menu

More formally, however, most intervention for autism has generally tended to sit in one of three categories: education, behaviour or medication. The focus has been on strategies which either aid adaptation to the issues that

> Interventions for autism have focused on education, behaviour and medication

autism brings, reduce the more challenging aspects and/or improve quality of life. An ideal intervention is one which perhaps crosses all three areas. Needless to say whole books have been written about these categories of intervention including a range of associated issues such as inclusive vs. specialised education, the best and worst ways to bring about behavioural changes and weighing up the effects of medicines on specific traits alongside their all important side-effects. All interventions have their proponents and their doubters. Importantly, there is seemingly no one-size-fits-all intervention for everyone with autism.

In recent years, discussions have also turned to questions about outcome following intervention. That is, questions about how useful early intervention might be over a lifetime, under what circumstances a 'reduction' in the symptoms of autism can occur and, indeed, whether reducing autistic symptoms and traits actually improves quality of life. These are not easy questions to answer given that we still know so little about the lifetime course of autism and what changes actually make a difference to someone not only having daily life skills but also obtaining employment, being financially and socially independent and if so desired, having a family life.

One final question to also think about: does intervention act directly on autism, or does it act on comorbidity which then acts on the presentation of autism? We'll be coming back to this question later on.

Don't mention those words

One of the more contentious issues under the intervention banner for autism is the use of the words 'cure' or 'recovery'. We're sure anyone who has ever searched the Internet for anything autism–related will have come across descriptions and accounts of people who had autism and are reported not to have autism anymore. The reasons for such accounts include just about every intervention that has ever been suggested for autism, often complete with an 'expert' to back up the claims. In research circles, talk of remedying autism has generally been met with a scientific scowl. Autism is a lifelong condition and no matter what intervention was in place, it wasn't something that people just grew out of in the same way that a person outgrows a pair of shoes. And those that said otherwise were ostracised.

With the growing consensus that autism is more accurately represented as the autisms, recent times have seen a subtle change in research attitudes to the idea that autism or at least the diagnosis of autism might not

> Some people with autism have been described as losing their symptoms (optimal outcome)

be as stable as once suggested. Emerging research on the possibility of different developmental trajectories[54] in relation to autism provided some of the impetus for people to start questioning the dogma of autism being a lifelong condition for everyone affected. First there were bloomers (developmental, not the underwear variety) and then the findings of one group which suggested the notion of **optimal outcome** in relation to specific cases of autism.[55] Said optimal outcome documented a group of children who were historically diagnosed as being on the autism spectrum, but for whatever reasons, moved outside of the diagnostic enclosure at follow-up. Autism science was excited.[56]

Before we get too ahead of ourselves and save any charges of giving a false image of autism for the majority of people, much more investigation is needed in the area of optimal outcome and developmental bloomers. Precise details on those who moved out of the autism spectrum and importantly what marks them as different from those where autism is a lifelong condition are still missing. Cases of natural remission from autism are still quite rare and questions arise as to the art form that is autism diagnosis.

Changing brain functions

Allied to all the talk about diagnostic instability in specific cases of autism are other emerging data focused on intervention and the potential benefits of early intervention with a view not just on behavioural changes but also more physiological changes. It is perhaps implied that any intervention for autism, where it works, has to be impacting on brain function somewhere along the way given the correlation with overt behaviours. Intervention for autism in the early years is generally taken to be more advantageous over later intervention given the perceived malleability of the growing brain in infancy and childhood compared with later ages (acknowledging that brain development is present throughout the lifespan).

> Early intervention may have the ability to affect brain function and development

As suggested in our brief discussion on the growing application of neuroscience to autism research, the tools of the neuroscience trade have seen significant advancement in terms of analytical and imaging power hinting at the inner workings of the brain. It is, therefore, unsurprising that investigations have started to look at both behavioural and neurological outcomes following intervention. A seminal paper by Dawson and colleagues[57] provided a tantalising insight into how one specific early behavioural intervention program might impact on brain activity. Focusing specifically on analyses of **electroencephalography (EEG)**– a technique normally used to diagnose specific types of epilepsy – the authors reported physiological changes correlating to the way the group in receipt of intervention processed faces post intervention. As preliminary as these results are, and accepting the requirement for quite a lot more replication, they do suggest that intervention might impact more broadly than just on observed behaviour.

Heterogeneity and comorbidity: the rule not the exception

In reaching the end of this chapter, you're probably starting to see a few common threads appearing about the nature of autism. That the label of autism represents a quite diverse range of presentations and functions should already be pretty evident. All this diversity is further complicated by some elevated risk for various developmental conditions also co-occurring alongside autism. The fact that combined heterogeneity and comorbidity do not lend themselves well to grand theories of autism and its nature is something that quite a few sciences involved in autism research have taken some years to work out. More focused research on smaller parts of the essence of the autism spectrum seems to be a primary way forward. Moreover, intervention, whilst not necessarily the same for everyone, might be doing much more than we originally thought.

> Autism is characterised by wide variation in presented symptoms and elevated risk of comorbidity

One small point that we need to make is that we have, on purpose, not included any detailed discussion about intellectual or **learning disability** as also occurring in cases of autism. It does occur, by the way, and in anywhere up to about 40 per cent of cases. We did this partly because we would have enough material to write another book on this topic. Also because there is still some degree of confusion as to whether one is able to make a definite distinction between what is autism and what is a specific categorical condition of intellectual disability outside of just using IQ as a determinant. In short, it's complicated.

In the next chapter, we're going to look at some of the other features and issues which can be present in cases of autism. You'll be happy to know that we are actually going to starting mentioning the words 'food' and 'diet' more as part of the conversation too.

References

36. Sasson NJ. *et al.* Autism and the broad autism phenotype: familial patterns and intergenerational transmission. *J Neurodev Disord.* 2013; 5: 11.
37. Gillberg C. The ESSENCE in child psychiatry: Early Symptomatic Syndromes Eliciting Neurodevelopmental Clinical Examinations. *Res Dev Disabil.* 2010; 31: 1543–1551.
38. Bolton PF. *et al.* Epilepsy in autism: features and correlates. *Br J Psychiatr.* 2011; 198: 289–294.
39. Hanson E. *et al.* Prevalence of Attention Deficit/Hyperactivity Disorder among individuals with an autism spectrum disorder. *J Autism Dev Disord.* 2012; Oct 13.
40. Cross-Disorder Group of the Psychiatric Genomics Consortium. Identification of risk loci with shared effects on five major psychiatric disorders: a genome-wide analysis. *Lancet.* 2013; 381:1371–1379.
41. Cuthbert BN. & Insel T. Toward the future of psychiatric diagnosis: the seven pillars of RDoC. *BMC Medicine* 2013; 11: 126.
42. Rutter M. Childhood schizophrenia reconsidered. *J Autism Child Schizophr.* 1972; 2: 315–337.
43. Unenge Hallerbäck M. *et al.* Is autism spectrum disorder common in schizophrenia? *Psychiatry Res.* 2012; 198: 12–17.

44. Gadow KD. Schizophrenia spectrum and attention-deficit/hyperactivity disorder symptoms in autism spectrum disorder and controls. *J Am Acad Child Adolesc Psychiatry*. 2012; 51: 1076–1084.
45. Davidson C. *et al.* Prevalence of Asperger syndrome among patients of an Early Intervention in Psychosis team. *Early Interv Psychiatry*. March 2013. DOI: 10.1111/eip.12039.
46. Catalá-López F. *et al.* Prevalence of attention deficit hyperactivity disorder among children and adolescents in Spain: a systematic review and meta-analysis of epidemiological studies. *BMC Psychiatry*. 2012; 12: 168.
47. Thapar A. *et al.* What have we learnt about the causes of ADHD? *J Child Psychol Psychiatry*. 2013; 54: 3–16.
48. Sinzig J. *et al.* Attention deficit/hyperactivity disorder in children and adolescents with autism spectrum disorder: symptom or syndrome? *J Atten Disord*. 2009; 13: 117–126.
49. Shen H. Blog post: *Neuroscientists brainstorm goals for US brain-mapping initiative*. Nature News. 2013. http://blogs.nature.com/news/2013/05/neuroscientists-brainstorm-goals-for-us-brain-mapping-initiative.html
50. Bettelheim B. The *empty fortress: infantile autism and the birth of the self*. The Free Press. New York. 1967
51. Happé F. *et al.* Time to give up on a single explanation for autism. *Nat Neurosci*. 2006; 9: 1218–1220.
52. Baron-Cohen S. *et al.* Does the autistic child have a "theory of mind"? *Cognition*. 1985; 21: 37–46.
53. Kagohara DM. *et al.* Using iPods(®) and iPads(®) in teaching programs for individuals with developmental disabilities: a systematic review. *Res Dev Disabil*. 2013; 34: 147–156.
54. Fountain C. *et al.* Six developmental trajectories characterize children with autism. *Pediatrics*. 2012; 129: e11121120.
55. Fein D. *et al.* Optimal outcome in individuals with a history of autism. *J Child Psychol Psychiatry*. 2013; 54: 195–205.
56. Ozonoff S. Editorial: Recovery from autism spectrum disorder (ASD) and the science of hope. *J Child Psychol Psychiatry*. 2013; 54: 113–114.
57. Dawson G. *et al.* Early behavioral intervention is associated with normalized brain activity in young children with autism. *J Am Acad Child Adolesc Psychiatry*. 2012; 51: 1150–1159.

RECIPES

Peppered mackerel fishcakes

A great way to introduce oily fish to children, these can be made in larger batches and frozen before you reach the cooking stage (serves 4).

Ingredients

1 small bunch of spring onions
4 medium potatoes
2 peppered mackerel fillets or 1 tin
1 egg
Fresh tarragon (if possible) or 1 tablespoon of dried tarragon
1 teaspoon of smoked paprika
Gluten-free plain flour
Olive oil for cooking

Method

Cut the spring onions into small pieces and place them in a bowl. Peel, cook and mash the potatoes and allow to cool. Break the mackerel into smaller pieces. Crack the egg into a small jug and whisk. Roughly chop the tarragon. Add the pieces of mackerel, mashed potatoes and paprika to the spring onions and stir in the tarragon. Put some flour on to your hands then form balls with the mixture, pat down into thick disks. Add olive oil to a pan and add the fish cakes and gently fry for 3 minutes on each side until golden brown. Serve hot with salad.

Sprinkling of nutritional science

The herb tarragon works well with many dishes but particularly those using fish. As one of the four king herbs of French cuisine, evidence is emerging that tarragon may well have appetite stimulating properties making it a potentially useful accompaniment in cases of problem eating.

Salmon tikka masala

A full–of–flavour quick curry (serves 4)

Ingredients

1 red chili
1 thumb size of fresh ginger
2 cloves of garlic
1 onion
1 green pepper
1 red pepper
2 tablespoons of olive oil
1 teaspoon of garam masala
1 teaspoon of turmeric

½ teaspoon of chili powder
1 tablespoon of tomato purée
4 salmon fillets
1 tin of chopped tomatoes
1 teaspoon of dairy-free spread
Juice of 1 lemon
2 tablespoon of fresh coriander

Method

Chop, grate or process the chili, ginger and garlic. Peel and roughly chop the onion. Cut the peppers into chunks. Cut the salmon into chunks. Heat up the olive oil in a frying pan. Add the chili, garlic, ginger and onion. Cook for 5 minutes. Add the spices and tomato purée and cook for 1 minute. Stir in the salmon and peppers and cook for 1 minute. Add the chopped tomatoes, bring to the boil and simmer for 10 minutes. Add the dairy-free spread and squeeze in the lemon last minute and stir. Garnish with coriander and serve with some rice.

Sprinkling of nutritional science

Coriander leaves are the perfect herbal accompaniment to many dishes with their strong taste. As with many other herbs and spices, coriander is a great source of antioxidants. It is with reference to its antibacterial activity though that there is some scientific interest in coriander oil and the wide range of bacteria which might be affected by its use.

Salmon fillet with garlic mash and mango, strawberry and coriander salsa

This fruity salsa adds a sweet zing to the salmon and boiling the garlic gives the mash a background flavour (serves 4).

Ingredients

4 thick-cut salmon fillets
1 tablespoon of groundnut oil
1 tablespoon of roast sesame oil
Salt and pepper to taste

For the salsa
1 medium green chili, finely chopped
1 medium red onion, peeled and finely diced
1 medium mango, skin and stone removed, then finely diced
200g strawberries, hulled and finely chopped
1 large handful coriander
1 tablespoon sherry vinegar
Juice of ½ lime

For the garlic mash
400g of floury potatoes, peeled and diced
5 cloves garlic, peeled
Salt and pepper to taste

Method

For the salsa, prepare all the ingredients and combine in a bowl. Leave to rest and infuse in the fridge until ready to serve. Cook the potatoes and garlic in salt water until tender. Mash with a potato masher or ricer, adjust seasoning. Keep warm until ready to serve. Pan-fry the salmon in the oils, skin down first, until starting to brown but still pink in the middle. Season while it cooks. Turn over and fry on the flesh side for another 2 or 3 minutes. Assemble on plates by placing a pile of garlic mash in the middle, lay the salmon fillet on top and spoon the salsa around. Serve with some salad, if you like.

Sprinkling of nutritional science

The mango – the national fruit of several countries including India – is a versatile fruit which can be used as part of both sweet and savoury dishes. A good source of various **vitamins** and **minerals** including vitamin A, important for eye health, mangoes contain various polyphenols and carotenoids, important for maintaining good health.

Chapter 3

The add-ons

When Dr Leo Kanner published what is widely credited as the first formal descriptions of autism in 1943[31] he perhaps unknowingly set the tone for how autism was to be viewed for decades to come. His descriptions – based on his training and occupation in psychiatry – talked in the most part about the overt behaviours he observed: behaviour not only of the 11 children who presented at his clinic but also observations about their parents, and the many and varied comments he made about them in his original manuscript. Some might argue that these comments about the mothers and fathers, whether taken in or out of context, helped play a role in the shaping and proliferation of a period of autism research history based on the prevailing psychogenic ideas of the time[50]. Kanner subsequently rejected any notion of attributing parental blame.

Outside of detailing what eventually became the triad of impairments – now boiled down to a dyad in at least one interpretation – several other important observations were made by Kanner. He described, for example, how several children in his case series presented with feeding difficulties including early vomiting and how some children had to be tube-fed during early infancy. He also remarked that several children showed motor issues; that is, problems with walking and movement.

Whilst the core features he described have long been taken up into diagnostic texts to separate autism from not-autism, some of his other, potentially important, observations were seemingly left as mere coincidental artefacts of his caseload. Whether this was due to his initial focus on observable behaviour or down to the way various disciplines have subsequently claimed the label of autism, one cannot help but think how different things might have been if other branches of medicine had first described autism. Say, for example, someone like Dr Asbjörn Fölling who discovered the archetypal 'diet can influence behaviour' inborn error of metabolism, **phenylketonuria (PKU) in 1934** – one of the conditions tested for as part of those few drops of blood taken from every infant.

Whilst we are in no way questioning the core commonalities which we now see as the diagnostic criteria for autism, in the context of the rise of the 'autisms' one could speculate that those artefacts reported by Kanner may not be as coincidental as perhaps indicated. Indeed based on the recent focus on **comorbidity** and how the description of comorbidity might surpass just the diagnostic labels that we assign and use, we could argue that chance artefacts should never be seen simply as chance artefacts but rather something rather more integral to the presentation of autism in a person.

I sense something

Whilst we hope that this book will live up to readers' expectations and offer pertinent information on our chosen topic area, we have to accept that in relation to some aspects of autism we are merely observers looking in. Take for example, the quite voluminous literature reporting on the various sensory and perceptual issues present in cases of autism.[58] It would be easy to quote study after study detailing this or that aspect of how people with autism perceive the world and list them rote fashion.

> Sensory issues affecting how the world is perceived have been frequently reported in autism

But, unlike detailing whether someone has spoken language or partakes in eye contact or not in a particular situation, the individual experiences of sensation and perception are never going to be something that can easily described with any great deal of accuracy. If you don't believe us, have a bite of that chocolate bar you have hidden in your cupboard and tell us exactly what it tastes like (and don't just describe it as 'chocolatey'). Even better describe to us the sound of Elvis Presley's voice, or how the inside of your car smells today. It's difficult isn't it? That and the fact that chocolate to you might taste very different to us individually and so on.

You'll probably already be familiar with the five traditional senses: vision, hearing, smell, taste and touch. We rely on these senses every second of our waking day to feed us information about our surroundings. Coupling them with other sensations like pain and temperature, we build and maintain a dynamic representation of ourselves and our current position in the world, or least our brain does, in its job of making sense of all those incoming signals and information.

The range of sensory issues described as being present in autism is wide. Ranging from descriptions of children with a pre-diagnosis of autism who were thought to be hearing impaired because they did not respond to questions or instructions, through to experiences with the use of Irlen lenses and coloured overlays to help alleviate issues like scotopic sensitivity syndrome (please look it up), multiple examples are available. Indeed, as part of the new clinical definition of **DSM-5**, such issues are no longer just comorbidity but something altogether more central to autism.

As we write, there is no one-size-fits-all standard when it comes to sensory-perceptual issues linked to autism, just as there isn't when it comes to not-autism. It does appear however that quite a few people on the autism spectrum are sensitive to certain types of perceptual information whether in amount or from specific origins. The terms 'hyposensitive' and 'hypersensitive', denoting higher or lower thresholds for receiving sensory information, are quite often used.

Now we're motoring

Perhaps one of the most under-rated group of people who become involved in the lives and care of people with autism are the **occupational therapists** or **OTs**. As the archetypal all-rounder, the areas which they can consult on are truly wide-ranging and often have an immediate impact on day-to-day living for lots of different groups of people. One area which occupational therapy certainly can and does impact upon is in relation to movement disorders.

Although Kanner may have to some extent downplayed the various coincidental features of movement irregularities present in his case series, the representation of such issues in autism in more modern times has been more accommodating. The spectrum of motor impairments reported alongside cases of autism is deserving of an entire book of its own given that a range of fine and gross motor skills – differentiating between those smaller and larger physical actions – have been reported as being problematic. Issues with gait and walking,[59] including specific types of behaviour such as toe walking,[60] through to handwriting skills[61] have all come under scrutiny with autism in mind. Indeed for some authors, motor coordination problems have also been suggested to be a 'cardinal feature' of autism[62] perhaps even with some diagnostic potential.[63]

> Problems with fine and gross motor skills can be present in autism

Anxious people

Stress and anxiety are common descriptions of modern-day life. Whether it is through juggling the work-life balance, or making sure there is food on the table and a roof over your head, we're all subject to the various strains of life. But does such common usage of a term like anxiety actually do justice to what it truly means to be chronically anxious?

Having previously alluded to some of the politics of autism and the use of the word 'disability' as one description, we turn our attention to the issues of stress and anxiety appearing alongside autism. Indeed, how often such manifestations are very correctly labelled as disability given their personal, social and even health-related effects on a person; in some cases, over and above the effects of the core symptoms of autism.

> Anxiety can be a big problem for people with autism, often severely affecting daily living

There is some good evidence to suggest that the way stress physically manifests in some people with autism is slightly different to that usually expected. Measurements of **cortisol** – an important hormone released under conditions of stress – are known to be elevated for some people with autism, even when taking into account the natural cycles and variations expected across different times of the day.[64] Perhaps of greater significance are the suggestions that still after a stress-inducing event has passed, measured cortisol levels in cases of autism might not necessarily decrease with as much urgency as observed in other groups of people.[65] Whilst still subject to further investigation, the notion of a perseverance of the heightened state of stress in autism offers potentially important clues to account for other peripheral features which can accompany autism (tantrums, meltdowns) and how they can manifest and persist.

Anxiety presenting alongside autism can occur for lots of different reasons. There is no doubt that what stresses us is more than likely going to stress someone with autism too. That being said, if one takes into account issues like the preoccupations a person may have (potentially bordering on conditions like obsessive-compulsive disorder) or perhaps a fear of new or novel situations, places, etc., added to some degree of social anxiety, it can perhaps be envisaged how anxiety might be a more frequent visitor for some people on the autism spectrum. And to reiterate, it can be utterly disabling.

Aggression

When talking about aggression in the context of autism, either directed towards others or indeed self-directed aggression or self-injurious behaviour, one has to bear a few things in mind. First and foremost is that whilst aggression is not a socially desirable response from anyone, we're all guilty of using it at some point in our lives whether diagnosed with autism or not. As children, aggression is often used as a way of communicating: '*that's my toy not yours*', often followed by the sound of fighting and crying, and is just one example. One might even argue that the whole activity of rough-and-tumble play with the emphasis on 'rough' is yet another manifestation of aggression and how it is a part of growing up and learning how to communicate.

Second is the quite sensitive issue of how aggression is portrayed in the case of autism and its wide spectrum of presentation, alongside all that elevated risk of comorbidity. Recent years have seen several incidents whereby dreadful events carried out by individuals against others have focused attention on issues like aggression and dangerousness in relation to segments of the autism spectrum. In the most part, the discussions after such incidents have very sensibly concentrated on the individual perpetrator and their own motivations and intentions, over and above any sweeping generalisations. But like the example of **schizophrenia** and dangerousness, and how it is portrayed by some, there is always the fear of stigma setting in, distorting and generalising without appropriate supporting evidence.

Bearing these points in mind, it would be neglectful if we were not to talk about aggression as being part of the presentation of autism for some. Although it is difficult to ascertain an accurate figure for how prevalent aggression is, in all its forms, in cases of autism, estimates range anywhere from 20–50 per cent depending on the severity of autism and other comorbidity.[66] Indeed whilst not necessarily a perfect correlation, the severity of autism and presence of **comorbid intellectual disability** seems to show some link with the likelihood of aggression and related factors like irritability.

Outside of the limited body of literature discussing how aggression presented in cases of autism might bring individuals into contact with the criminal justice system, there are numerous accounts discussing how families and caregivers meet and have to cope with aggression from their loved ones

> Aggression – either to themselves or towards others – can occur in autism but does not mean people with autism are a danger to others

with autism. Accounts talk about children having tantrums and meltdown with associated aggressive outbursts perhaps tied into some of the previous factors we have just discussed. They also talk about children with autism growing up into tall and strong adults being cared for and managed by often ageing parents, and the challenges that brings particularly during transitional times such as the onset of puberty.

There are no straightforward answers as to why aggression, and particularly self-aggression, seems to appear in relation to autism. One might speculate that for those particularly lacking verbal speech as a communicative tool, aggression could be part of their language; for example, communicating emotions or pain and discomfort or indeed to block out even more painful issues such as headaches, toothaches or related issues. One might even view such behaviours as part of a coping strategy. It is even possible that aggression may be due to other more biologically based reasons.[67]

Medical comorbidity

Having introduced the finding that conditions like **ADHD** and schizophrenia can appear or coexist alongside autism, often with far greater frequency than would be typically expected, we turn to some of the other issues that have also been documented albeit with a more traditional physiological or somatic basis to them. Obviously we don't have the space to talk about every single finding reported in relation to autism so we are going to be a little bit selective in what we discuss. It is, however, important that we reiterate that a diagnosis of autism is seemingly protective of nothing when it comes to the possibility of developing other conditions or comorbidities whether psychiatric or physical.

The brain's electrics

Whilst autism is not generally thought to be a life-limiting condition, that's not to say that autism and its effects or risk of comorbidity are not sometimes implicated in early mortality. Much recent focus has

> Epilepsy or seizure disorder can occur alongside autism and requires due attention and care

turned to the issue of wandering in relation to autism[68] and the sometimes devastating outcome such episodes can lead to. As terrible as such accounts are, wandering is not what would be described as a leading cause of early death for people with autism. Death as a consequence of epilepsy or a seizure might, however, have the dubious honour of a more prominent place in any list of causes.[69]

There are unfortunately very few, if any, positive things to say about epilepsy. As well as being implicated in early death it is a condition, or rather group of conditions, which needs care and management often for years or a lifetime. That's not to say that people with epilepsy can't live a normal life. With advances in medicines and other available techniques, many are successful in controlling their epilepsy.

Autism has a grim link with epilepsy. It has been estimated that anywhere between 5 and 40 per cent of people with autism will develop some form of epilepsy over a lifetime,[70] far in excess of the risk to the general population. Having previously talked about the difficulties in disentangling autism from a specific diagnosis of **intellectual disability (ID)**, it does appear that the presence of ID or not can be a moderating factor in the risk of onset.[71]

Look to the eyes

Although sensory-perceptual issues are sometimes a part of the presentation of autism, it would be wrong to assume that there might not be underlying medical reasons to account for such observations. Take

> Eye problems affecting vision and perception can occur alongside autism

for example, the research reported by Ikeda and colleagues.[72] Based on their patient audit, they suggested that upwards of 40 per cent of people with autism in their group had ophthalmologic pathology; that is a specific medical condition related to their eyes potentially affecting visual function. Allowing for the potential difficulties in assessing for such visual problems, particularly for those with a more severe presentation of autism who may not be verbally responsive to questions and queries, there are important implications from such a finding. Primary is whether such physical issues might, in some part, be contributory to the sensory or indeed other behaviours reported by some people on the autism spectrum.

Lifestyle diseases

The theme of health inequality being increasingly recognised as appearing alongside conditions like schizophrenia[73] might also be a point of further investigation in relation to autism. Specifically, the increasing recognition that autism is not protective against the development of various lifestyle related conditions such as obesity and other features of the so-called **metabolic syndrome** (elevated **cholesterol**, blood sugar, blood pressure, etc.) and their subsequent impact on heart disease, **diabetes** and stroke.

> People with autism are just as likely to present with obesity or diabetes as the rest of the population

Various estimates indicate that people with autism are at least as likely to present as clinically obese as those in the general population.[74] Insofar as conditions like diabetes are characterised by problems in controlling blood sugar levels, there is some evidence pointing towards a potential connection between autism and type-1 diabetes over type-2 diabetes[75] also suggesting some involvement for **autoimmunity** in relation to cases. Cholesterol levels, and their correlations in relation to health and disease, are still subject to some discussions in the wider health circle. There do not seem to be any definitive trends to the current data with autism in mind. Some studies have reported signs of dyslipidemia – abnormal lipid levels – in cases of autism[76]; others have conversely reported lower cholesterol levels to be present.[77] Indeed, drawing on the work looking at the significant presence of autism or autistic traits in cases of Smith-Lemli-Opitz syndrome (SLOS)[78] a condition characterised by malfunction in the ability to make cholesterol, one can see how much greater investigation is required in this area.

Powerhouse

Some readers may have heard use of the term **mitochondria** with reference to some cases of autism. Probably the best description of mitochondria (plural of mitochondrion) in relation to their primary function is power; the power they provide to cells. Although outside the scope of this book, the relationship between mitochondria and autism, controversial at times,[79] is still the source of some discussion given the wide-ranging findings that have been reported. Interested readers are advised to read the excellent paper by Rossignol and Frye[80] for a more authoritative review and overview of this area of autism research.

> Mitochondrial issues affecting cell functions have been reported in several cases of autism

Several individual findings are worthy of mention with mitochondria in mind including those related to elevations in plasma lactate levels[81] and issues with the acylcarnitines.[82] You guessed it though, more research is needed.

The selection of more medical/physiology-based comorbidity that we have provided, whilst not exhaustive, reiterates how autism is not a stand-alone condition. Further it suggests that there may be some possible interconnectedness of some of the add-on symptoms we have described. We'll be looking further at this idea later in the book. Ensuring that at least part of this book will talk about diet and autism has not given us the opportunity to explore various other conditions also reported as being present in cases of autism either in the research literature or more informally. If any reader is interested, we could suggest looking up the various discussions on things like sleeping issues, joint hypermobility, and even **chronic fatigue syndrome/myalgic encephalomyelitis (CFS/ME)**. Of course, we're not necessarily suggesting that these conditions are going to feature in every case of autism; merely that autism seemingly offers no protection against such issues. Oh, and if you think we missed out one particular area related to our deepest, darkest recesses, namely talk of toilets and 'number twos', that's all coming up in the next chapter.

References

58. Donnellan AM. *et al.* Rethinking autism: implications of sensory and movement differences for understanding and support. *Front Integr Neurosci.* 2012; 6: 124.
59. Chester VL. and Calhoun M. Gait symmetry in children with autism. *Autism Res Treat.* 2012; 2012: 576478.
60. Barrow WJ. *et al.* Persistent toe walking in autism. *J Child Neurol.* 2011; 26: 619–621.
61. Fuentes CT. *et al.* Children with autism show specific handwriting impairments. *Neurology.* 2009; 73: 1532–1537.
62. Fournier KA. *et al.* Motor coordination in autism spectrum disorders: a synthesis and meta-analysis. *J Autism Dev Disord.* 2010; 40: 1227–1240.
63. Green D. *et al.* The severity and nature of motor impairment in Asperger's syndrome: a comparison with specific developmental disorder of motor function. *J Child Psychol Psychiatry.* 2002; 43: 655–668.
64. Kidd SA. *et al.* Daytime secretion of salivary cortisol and alpha-amylase in preschool-aged children with autism and typically developing children. *J Autism Dev Disord.* 2012; 42: 2648–2658.
65. Spratt EG. *et al.* Enhanced cortisol response to stress in children in autism. *J Autism Dev Disord.* 2012; 42: 75–81.
66. Richards C. *et al.* Self-injurious behaviour in individuals with autism spectrum disorder and intellectual disability. *J Intellect Disabil Res.* 2012; 56: 476–489.
67. Hof PR. *et al.* Neuropathological observations in a case of autism presenting with self-injury behavior. *Acta Neuropathol.* 1991; 82: 321–326.
68. Anderson C. *et al.* Occurrence and family impact of elopement in children with autism spectrum disorders. *Pediatrics.* 2012; 130: 870–877.
69. Bilder D. *et al.* Excess mortality and causes of death in autism spectrum disorders: a follow up of the 1980s Utah/UCLA autism epidemiologic study. *J Autism Dev Disord.* 2013; 43: 1196–1204.
70. Tuchman R. & Rapin I. Epilepsy in autism. *Lancet Neurol.* 2002; 1: 352–358.
71. Berg AT. & Plioplys S. Epilepsy and autism: is there a special relationship? *Epilepsy Behav.* 2012; 23: 193–198.
72. Ikeda J. *et al.* Brief report: Incidence of ophthalmologic disorders in children with autism. *J Autism Dev Disord.* February 2012.
73. Subashini R. *et al.* Prevalence of diabetes, obesity, and metabolic syndrome in subjects with and without schizophrenia (CURES-104). *J Postgrad Med.* 2011; 57: 272–277.
74. Curtin C. *et al.* The prevalence of obesity in children with autism: a secondary data analysis using nationally representative data from the National Survey of Children's Health. *BMC Pediatr.* 2010; 10: 11.
75. Freeman SJ. *et al.* Type 1 diabetes and autism: is there a link? *Diabetes Care.* 2005; 28: 925–926.
76. Dziobek I. *et al.* Hypercholesterolemia in Asperger syndrome: independence from lifestyle, obsessive-compulsive behavior, and social anxiety. *Psychiatry Res.* 2007; 149: 321–324.

77. Tierney E. *et al*. Abnormalities of cholesterol metabolism in autism spectrum disorders. *Am J Med Genet B Neuropsychiatr Genet*. 2006; 141B: 666–668.
78. Sikora DM. *et al*. The near universal presence of autism spectrum disorders in children with Smith-Lemli-Opitz syndrome. *Am J Med Genet A*. 2006; 140: 1511–1518.
79. Offit PA. Vaccines and autism revisited—the Hannah Poling case. *N Engl J Med*. 2008; 358: 2089–2091.
80. Rossignol DA. & Frye RE. Mitochondrial dysfunction in autism spectrum disorders: a systematic review and meta-analysis. *Mol Psychiatry*. 2012; 17: 290–314.
81. Oliveira G. *et al*. Mitochondrial dysfunction in autism spectrum disorders: a population-based study. *Dev Med Child Neurol*. 2005; 47: 185–189.
82. Frye RE. *et al*. Unique acyl-carnitine profiles are potential biomarkers for acquired mitochondrial disease in autism spectrum disorder. *Transl Psychiatry*. 2013; 3: e220.

RECIPES

Roasted chickpeas

A handy snack for on the go, you can experiment with the spices and herbs

Ingredients

One tin of chickpeas
¼ teaspoon of salt (or to taste)
½ teaspoon of garlic powder
½ teaspoon of smoked paprika

Method

Preheat the oven to 200 degrees centigrade / 180 degrees centigrade for a fan oven / gas mark 6. Toss the chickpeas, salt, and spices together in a small bowl until the chickpeas are all evenly coated. Place a silicon baking sheet or baking parchment on to a baking tray and spread the chickpeas evenly. Bake for 45–60 minutes; stirring every 15 minutes for even cooking, until they become hard and crunchy. Store in an airtight container for up to a week

Sprinkling of nutritional science

Chickpeas have a long history as a food source. A good source of **folic acid** and zinc, chickpeas are packed with protein and low in fat.

Pear, pecan and pancetta salad

Sweet, crunchy and salty combo; you should be able to find pomegranate molasses in larger supermarkets

Ingredients per person

2 slices of pancetta
½ ripe pear
1 celery stick
Small handful candied pecans
1 small cereal bowl of mixed leaves such as rocket, watercress, spinach
1 tablespoon pomegranate molasses

How to candy pecans

Add the pecans to a small saucepan with 2 tablespoons of sugar and 2 tablespoons of water. Stir to dissolve the sugar and bring to a boil. Immediately turn down the heat to simmer for 5–7 minutes. Keep an eye on them as they are easily burnt. The syrup should be mostly gone or the pecans will be too sticky. Place them on some parchment or baking paper to cool. These can be stored in an airtight container.

Method

In a frying or griddle pan crisp the pancetta, place on some kitchen paper to absorb the excess fat. With a knife, quarter the pear, remove the core (you can peel if you wish) and slice into 3mm thick pieces. Slice the celery in to similarly sized pieces and mix with the leaves and pear. Drizzle with the pomegranate molasses and toss together then scatter with the nuts and top with the pancetta.

Sprinkling of nutritional science

Think spinach and most people will think of the character Popeye and his yearning for the green stuff. Indeed Popeye may very well have been right to include spinach in his diet as those leaves pack a mighty nutritional punch ounce for ounce containing high levels of **vitamin** K, vitamin C, folic acid and **iron**.

Homemade bouillon

Stock up on your stock; ready to go in any casserole, curry, stew or soup

Ingredients

100 grams of fennel bulb, chopped
100 grams of carrots, well scrubbed and chopped
100 grams of celery
75 grams of leeks, sliced and well washed
100 grams of fine grain sea salt
Black pepper corns, crushed
30 grams of sun-dried tomatoes
100 grams of onion, peeled
3 medium garlic cloves
30 grams of dried porcini mushrooms
40 grams of flat-leaf parsley, roughly chopped
40 grams of dill, roughly chopped

Method

Place the fennel, carrot, celery and leek in a food processor and pulse, add the rest of the ingredients and pulse again; you may need to move the ingredients about to ensure all the ingredients are evenly chopped. You should end up with a loose paste. Place in an airtight jar and store in the freezer. Due to the salt in the mixture it will stay scoopable. You could also make this mixture without salt and freeze into ice cube trays to allow seasoning to taste of each dish.

Suggested use

Use 1 teaspoon per 250ml of liquid

Sprinkling of nutritional science

Mushrooms are in effect the fruit of a fungus. They come in all shapes and sizes as well as different varieties possessing different chemical properties (not all good, it has to be said).

As well as being a good source of protein, the various edible mushrooms have been suggested to confer various health benefits including possessing immune-stimulating properties as a result of compounds such as beta-glucan. Beta-glucan present in grains such as oats has also been suggested to demonstrate cholesterol-lowering properties. Mushrooms are also thought to be a good source of selenium and other trace vitamins and **minerals**, including **vitamin D2**, vital for a healthy body.

Chicken curry with garlic green beans and spicy cauliflower nuggets

Aromatic, fantastic textures . . . packed with flavours (serves 4)

Chicken curry

Ingredients

2 tablespoons of vegetable oil
1 small onion, grated
2 cloves of garlic, chopped
4 skinless chicken breasts
3 teaspoons of ground turmeric
2 teaspoons of chili powder
1 (400g) tin chopped tomatoes
1 heaped teaspoon of bouillon paste (see previous recipe)/GF stock cube
1 tablespoon of dairy-free spread (optional)
3 teaspoons of ground cumin
3 teaspoons of ground coriander
2 tablespoons of grated fresh root ginger
1 tablespoon of chopped coriander leaves to garnish

Method

Heat the oil in a large deep pan. Add the onion and cook on a gentle heat for 10 minutes until softened. Add the garlic and cook for a further 2 minutes. Add the chicken, turmeric and chili powder. Fry gently, scraping the bottom of the pan frequently and turning the chicken. Add the tinned tomatoes, cover the pan, and simmer over a medium heat for 10 minutes. Uncover, and simmer for another 10 minutes to allow the liquid to reduce down. Add the bouillon, butter, cumin, ground coriander and ginger, and simmer for another 5 minutes. Serve with fresh coriander as a garnish.

Spicy cauliflower nuggets

Ingredients

1 large head of cauliflower
¼ cup of olive oil
1½ teaspoons of salt
1 teaspoon of black pepper

2 teaspoons of ground cumin
1 teaspoon of chili powder
1 teaspoon of paprika

Method

Preheat the oven to 200 degrees centigrade. Cut off and discard the stem of the cauliflower. Wash and cut up the cauliflower into small florets. In a large bowl, combine the olive oil, salt, pepper and spices together. Add the cauliflower pieces and thoroughly coat each piece. Place the cauliflower pieces on to a baking sheet lined with parchment paper. Bake for 1 hour and turn a few times during cooking until each piece has a nice brown colouring.

Garlic green beans

Ingredients

160 grams of green beans, topped and tailed then halved
2 garlic cloves, peeled
1 tablespoon of rapeseed or olive oil
½ teaspoon of chili flakes (optional)

Method

Steam the green beans for 3–5 minutes until cooked. Very finely slice the garlic. Heat the oil, add the garlic and allow to cook until the garlic begins to toast. Add the green beans and cook for a further 1 minute.

Sprinkling of nutritional science

As an alternative to other meat sources, chicken represents a great source of animal-derived protein as well as containing lots of other vitamins, minerals and essential **amino acids**. Whilst chicken is a great source of **tryptophan**, the starting material for **serotonin**, there is still some confusion as to how much tryptophan is absorbed in a useable form from the bird when eaten. Nonetheless, as a source of various B vitamins and being low in fat, chicken is a very versatile staple food source.

Thai chicken rice noodle soup
(Serves 4)

Ingredients

1 stalk of lemongrass, finely sliced and minced
3–4 kaffir lime leaves
1 thumb-size piece of ginger, grated or sliced into thin strips
3 cloves of garlic, minced
1 red chili, pierced all over with a knife
2–3 tablespoons of fish sauce (to taste)
1½ litres of chicken stock

1–2 fresh chicken breasts or thighs, chopped into small pieces, or 1–2 cups of leftover roast chicken
1 large carrot, peeled and finely ribboned using a peeler
Several bunches baby bok choi or pak choi
60 millilitres of fresh lime juice
1 teaspoon sugar (to taste)
Black pepper (to taste)
60 millilitres of coconut milk
200–250 grams of rice noodles
A large handful of fresh coriander to garnish

Method

In a large pan, place the lemongrass, ginger lime leaves, crushed garlic, whole chili, 2 tablespoons of fish sauce and chicken stock and bring to the boil over high heat. Add the chicken and cook for 5 minutes. Add the carrot and bok choi, lime juice, sugar and black pepper. Turn the heat down to a minimum and add the coconut milk and rice noodles and stir to incorporate. Taste-test the soup, adding more fish sauce, lime juice or sugar until you reach a suitable balance. If it tastes too salty, add another squeeze or two of lime juice. Serve with a final sprinkling of pepper and fresh coriander. You can top with chili sauce or oil for a spicier flavour if desired, serve with Thai chili sauce.

Sprinkling of nutritional science

Pak choi, also known as the Chinese cabbage, has long been used as a medicinal food. Aside from providing a very healthy serving of vitamin C, pak choi is low in fat and is a great source of fibre for aiding good gastrointestinal health.

Part II

The dietary science of autism

Chapter 4

All disease begins in the gut (and other sweeping generalisations)

We would like to apologise to readers for the title of this chapter. Throughout this book so far we've tried to emphasise how the currency of science is generally probability not absolutes and the allied notion of the plurality of autism. Then, here we go quoting Hippocrates, who it seems was more than a little obsessed with our inner workings in relation to health and disease and his seemingly very absolute opinion. In our defence, the point we were trying to make with the chapter title was that alongside the more usual processes that operate inside the human gastrointestinal (GI) tract or **gut**, there is an increasing body of scientific work linking its function and malfunction to a variety of GI and, seemingly non-GI centred conditions.

A description to start: picture if you will that long corridor stretching from our mouth to our, erm... other end, that is the gut. Even better, see the picture we've provided in Figure 4.1.

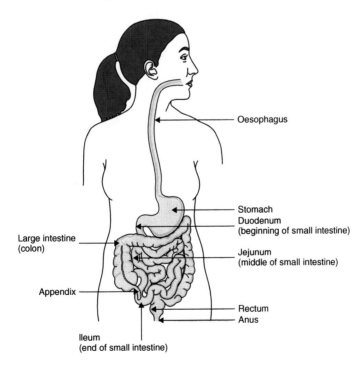

Figure 4.1 The gastrointestinal tract.

In between are the various biological systems which turn our food and drink into waste, hopefully along the way also allowing us to efficiently derive some life-sustaining nutrition from our various intakes. Without getting too technical, the main systems of the gut going from top to bottom are the **oesophagus**, the **stomach** and the large and small intestines (which themselves carry various sub-domains). Whilst all sounding relatively straightforward in design and function the gut is another marvel of biological engineering as a result of its astounding simplicity yet, at the same time, complexity. Little wonder that in some circles, it's talked about as being the second brain.[83]

The gut is alive. Not only because we are alive and the multitude of chemicals and **enzymes** that we produce exist and work in the gut, but also because of things like the mind-boggling numbers of bacteria and viruses that also inhabit our gut. The figures are astounding when you realise that of the trillions of bacteria which call us home – collectively known as the microbiome[84] – a sizable majority of them live in our gut. They dwarf the total numbers of cells present in the human body and are also seemingly involved in quite a few biological processes outside of the simple notion of merely aiding digestion.[85] Readers are forewarned that gut bacteria, the gut microbiota, feature quite heavily in our discussions on diet and autism.

> Trillions of bacteria live in our gastrointestinal (GI) tract and can affect our health

As suggested by that 'second brain' image, the gut also houses its own enteric nervous system complete with neurotransmitters. It's nothing like as complex as the brain in terms of number of neurons – the molecular transmitters – but it does mean that the gut can perform some of its duties on its own. Neurotransmitters such as **serotonin (5-HT)** and dopamine are also found in the gut. Indeed, surprisingly there is far more serotonin in the gut than there is in the brain which begs some interesting questions about whether our gut may play some role in our psychology given the link between serotonin and mood regulation.

It all sounds rather impressive doesn't it? Two brains in one body. Given then the importance and complexity of the gut, one can perhaps see how, when things go wrong with it, the consequences might be more far-reaching than just tummy problems.

Should we mention the gastrointestinal (GI) tract and autism?

Everyone, at some point in their lives, has an issue with their gut. It ranges from GI effects following infection or illness, as a result of taking various kinds of medicines, or as a result of the various food or liquids we drink. It's generally not polite conversation to bring up your problems 'downstairs', given that discussion more often than not turns to questions about your bowel productions, their frequency and consistency.

Having been in contact with several thousand families over the course of a research career in autism, at least one of the authors of this book knows how affectionately some parents talk about their child's stools. Some even have their own descriptions of said stools; to quote a colleague of ours, 'seat-lifters' and 'bog blockers', which we don't think need any further explanation. We use the word 'affectionately' to try and make easier the discussion of a topic which for some people on the autism spectrum has long been an integral part of their presentation. On a more serious note, such bowel issues can be the source of real pain and discomfort for some people with autism.

> Quite a few people with autism also have GI or bowel issues

It's a rather unfortunate truth in autism circles that some areas of discussion, debate and research have tended to stir up controversy and division. None more so than when talking about the gastrointestinal (GI) tract or the gut in relation to cases of autism. We're pretty sure that we don't need to mention the nature of these discussions, some of which have been quite widely publicised, and indeed modelled into one of Dr Insel's kingdoms of autism. We are going to explore some of the research into GI factors in cases of autism. Indeed given the focus of this book on a potential link between diet and cases of autism, one cannot fail to note that for any relationship to work between these two factors, one must assume the gut to be playing some kind of role.

The gut with the autism spectrum in mind has some research history going back to the 1960s and 1970s. Interestingly it was the father of **Asperger syndrome**, Hans Asperger, who was one of the first to bring to light a possible connection between the gut and the autism spectrum at least in some cases.[86] On that occasion he was talking about the extra-intestinal presentation of **coeliac disease** in children.

Coeliac disease

Since we've brought coeliac disease into the conversation we should perhaps pause the autism-gut conversation to talk about this very interesting condition and where it sits in the growing spectrum of diseases and disorders related to the protein **gluten**. Indeed, where it sits with autism in mind.

Coeliac disorder is an autoimmune condition. It's often misquoted as being an **allergy** to gluten, but the processes which have been uncovered so far suggest that it is not a simple case of the immune system mounting a traditional **IgE**-mediated response to gluten as normally happens in classical allergy. In essence, coeliac disease all starts with issues with metabolising gluten: the process of breaking the protein down.

Proteins are long chains of **amino acids**. Think of a very long pearl necklace as being something like gluten. Each pearl is one of its constituent amino acid. In order to metabolise the gluten necklace, our enzymes correctly functioning as a result of their **cofactors** go to work in the gut chopping up the protein necklace. Rather than, however, just exploding the protein into all its constituent pearls (amino acids), short chains of pearls are initially formed called **peptides**. Further digestion then takes place to work on these smaller peptides to eventually get at the nourishment, which is the individual amino acids.

In coeliac disease, that process of chopping up proteins to form those intermediate peptides actually produces peptides which don't want to be further digested by the body. These gluten epitopes, as they are also called, then gain access to a part of the gut

> Coeliac (celiac) disease is an autoimmune condition managed by following a gluten-free diet

lining or membrane called the lamina propria where their immunogenicity – the ability to provoke an immune response – is further increased by something called **tissue transglutaminase (tTG)**. It's then all about the immune system, or rather a servant of the immune system called the major histocompatability complex, which presents these modified peptides to the immune system. The body sees these peptides as foreign and accordingly mounts an immune response. That immune response involves the production of inflammatory **cytokines** – signalling molecules – among other things which leads to tissue damage of the gut mucosa. Said damage is characteristically illustrated by the flattened mucosa which leads to a malabsorptive state. It's quite a bit more complicated than our simple explanation suggests but there are plenty more detailed descriptions available.[87] Our diagram should also help.

Coeliac disease is a lifelong condition. It's estimated to affect approximately 1 per cent of the population although the accuracy of this figure is complicated by presentation and screening issues. Genetics plays a role in coeliac disease but, reflecting the crucial role that gluten ingestion plays in the presentation and perpetuation of the condition, the adoption of a gluten-free diet represents the first-line of treatment. Figure 4.2 shows some of the main mechanisms linked to coeliac disease.

Following the paper by Asperger, several efforts have been directed to examining the prevalence of coeliac disease in cases of autism. The results have not been overwhelming in demonstrating people with autism as being at elevated risk of coeliac disease over the population at large.[88] There have been reports suggesting, however, that screening for coeliac disease might be indicated when a diagnosis of autism is received.[89] That and specific elements of coeliac disease aetiology such as tTG antibody markers also being isolated in quite a few cases of autism[90] at least hinting at some propensity towards **autoimmunity** being implicated. Importantly, a diagnosis of autism does not seemingly protect against the risk of presenting with coeliac disease.

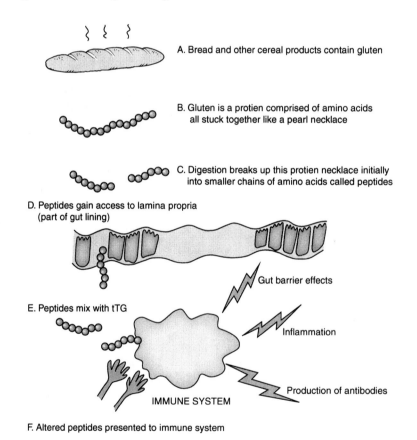

A. Bread and other cereal products contain gluten

B. Gluten is a protien comprised of amino acids all stuck together like a pearl necklace

C. Digestion breaks up this protien necklace initially into smaller chains of amino acids called peptides

D. Peptides gain access to lamina propria (part of gut lining)

Gut barrier effects

E. Peptides mix with tTG

Inflammation

Production of antibodies

IMMUNE SYSTEM

F. Altered peptides presented to immune system

Figure 4.2 Coeliac disease.

Before heading into the whole spectrum of gluten issues which more and more seems to be talked about, we'd like to drop in the case study presented by Genuis and Bouchard.[91] Whilst you might roll your eyes about our bringing up a case report, we might take you back to our previous discussions on **heterogeneity** and the potential value of the N=1 with autism in mind. Genuis and Bouchard described a case of a boy with autism and concurrent coeliac disease. The introduction of a gluten-free diet positively affected the presentation of coeliac disease but also that of the boy's autism. As coincidental as this description might be, within the context of evidence looking at neurological manifestations of coeliac disease as in, for instance, the collected works of Dr Marios Hadjivassiliou and colleagues[92] one might not necessarily consign such observations solely to chance or scientific bias.

> Studies have reported behavioural changes in cases of autism and coeliac disease following commencement of a gluten-free diet

Gluten issues: another spectrum?

Based on the available data, we can perhaps reject, or at least strongly challenge, any universal notion that autism appears as a result of undiagnosed coeliac disease. That's not to say that autism and coeliac disease can't coexist together however. Given also that coeliac disease is not widely tested for when an autism diagnosis is received, there may still be a pool of people with autism carrying the genetic and serological markers of the condition.

Whilst coeliac disease represents the archetypal 'gluten is a problem' condition, there is a revolution currently underway in the science of gluten sensitivity: a revolution which still maintains coeliac disease as a primary presentation of issues with gluten, but at the same time acknowledges that there may in fact be a spectrum of gluten-related disorders[93] including **non-coeliac gluten intolerance**.[94] At the time of writing, there is still much to do in terms of defining the gluten disorder spectrum and the core features linked to various manifestations. There are, however, some clues about which areas might provide defining and differentiating factors related to immune function and mucosal barrier function.[95]

General zonulin

One particularly interesting area of study is that related to a compound called **zonulin**. Whilst sounding like something from a sci-fi movie, zonulin is a protein of some potential note in various gut-related conditions given its gatekeeper role in relation to the gut membrane.[96] We'll be coming on to the gut barrier in more detail shortly, but in brief, zonulin is thought to be a primary factor in opening the spaces between cells in the gut allowing certain things like nutrients through whilst keeping harmful bacteria out.

Think zonulin and one name keeps cropping up: Dr Alessio Fasano, a pediatric gastroenterologist. His various studies on zonulin have demonstrated quite a robust link between zonulin and increased gut barrier permeability in various autoimmune conditions including type-1 **diabetes**[97] and coeliac disease.[98]

> Zonulin is a protein suggested to affect the permeability of the gaps between cells in the gut barrier

There is still much that is not known about zonulin and its barrier duties, not least the ways and means by which zonulin release and upregulation come about. There is a suggestion that gliadin, a part of gluten, can activate zonulin signalling and therefore increase gut barrier permeability.[99] Although only investigated on cell lines in the laboratory and so not necessarily charting the complexity of real life, the possibility that gluten may induce zonulin production and subsequently increase gut barrier permeability – **leaky gut** – might overlap with various other findings including those potentially related to cases of autism.

The great barrier and the leaky gut

We've gone and said it haven't we? Those words: leaky gut, and the images they conjure up of an old metal bucket dotted with holes leaking water everywhere. Even better, those old cartoons we saw as children with a certain cat and mouse and the funny after-effects of said cat drinking water subsequent to being perforated by something or other by the mouse.

Discuss leaky gut in some quarters of the scientific landscape and you'll get some interesting responses. The UK NHS Choices website entry[100] on 'leaky gut syndrome' for example, epitomises quite a typical response, with headings like 'Why we should be sceptical about "leaky gut syndrome"' and mention of 'alternative medicine'. The fact that they also propose that the promotion of the condition is just a way of selling 'diet books' might also raise an eyebrow. Just for the record, we didn't write this book on the back of some leaky gut craze. We're going to mention more about complementary/alternative medicine in future chapters so will leave that for now.

Leaky gut is actually a bit of a misnomer. Everyone has some degree of gut leakiness or permeability simply because we need to absorb nutrients from our food and allow said nutrients access to the wider body outside of just the gut. It is perhaps more accurate to describe a state or condition where increased intestinal permeability or gut hyperpermeability is present and persistent to illustrate the circumstances being discussed and the potential knock-on effects this might have (see Figure 4.3).

> Leaky gut describes a state of increased gut permeability potentially allowing food, chemicals or bacteria access to other parts of the body

The barrier which separates the contents of our gut from the beginnings of our immune system is surprisingly thin; only a single layer of epithelial cells. As in coeliac disease, when the barrier is breached it unleashes a whole cascade of immune effects which themselves have a negative effect on barrier integrity. One need only look at the example of sepsis – a state of widespread **inflammation** in response to an infection – where gut barrier function has been implicated as a function of bacterial translocation[101] to see how severe this can become. Bacterial translocation, by the way, refers to the notion of gut bacteria finding their way into other areas of the body by means of crossing the gut barrier and provoking an immune response. You'll hear more about this shortly.

The structure and integrity of those epithelial cells is governed by a group of compounds known collectively as the intercellular junctional complexes.[102] This complex is, in effect, the sealant of the gut barrier bridging the gap between cells. In contrast, however, to any ideas of bathroom sealants or related examples, the complex represents a dynamic group of compounds that are reactive to various interactions with bacteria and food for example.[103] Even psychological stress might play a role. **Tight junctions (TJ),**

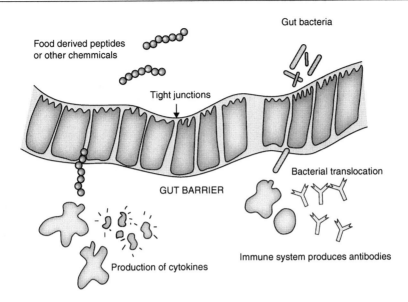

Figure 4.3 Leaky gut.

made up of various proteins, represent an important part of that complex regulating gut barrier integrity: that and their assembly or disassembly under various conditions.

We've already alluded to gut hyperpermeability potentially having a connection to autoimmune diseases in our mention of zonulin. Indeed, within the context of various autoimmune related conditions like type-1 diabetes, inflammatory bowel disease and coeliac disease, there seems to be some merit in further research and even the promise of potential new ways of symptom management being revealed.[104]

Autism and the leaky gut

Leaky gut or gut hyperpermeability has been proposed as a factor in cases of autism for some time. It's difficult to say precisely when gut hyperpermeability was first introduced into the autism literature but a best guess would be the seminal paper by Mary Goodwin and colleagues[105] very grandly titled: 'Malabsorption and cerebral dysfunction: a multi-variate and comparative study of autistic children'. In it, Goodwin and colleagues talked about, among other things, a gut–brain interface as potentially being relevant to cases of autism.

Complementary to that solitary case report on autism and coeliac disease detailed by Genuis and Bouchard[91], Goodwin and colleagues discussed their earlier findings[106] of how a gluten-free diet seemed to have more than just a physiological effect on a child diagnosed with coeliac disease and comorbid autism. Importantly, they reported effects following a gluten challenge, the reintroduction of gluten, and how it 'produced a brief relapse with exacerbation of autistic symptoms'. Again to reiterate, this was a case description.

The Goodwin paper was then followed by quite a long research pause on the topic of autism and gut permeability until 1996 and the published results from Patricia D'Eufemia and colleagues.[107] D'Eufemia *et al.* should perhaps hold the accolade as being the first group to actually measure gut permeability in relation to autism. Relying on the sugar intestinal permeability test (measuring recovery ratios of two sugars, mannitol and lactulose, in urine) they reported quite a high frequency of altered gut permeability (43 per cent) in their small cohort of children and young adults with autism. Interestingly, their results hinted that the nature of the permeability present may be more reflective of paracellular permeability which might imply 'some damage to tight junctions of the gut mucosa'.

Subsequent research, albeit limited in quantity, has also been reported with gut permeability measurement in mind. Contrasted with the D'Eufemia findings, Robertson and colleagues[108] reported no differences in sugar intestinal permeability test results in their cohort. Perhaps importantly for the most recent study by Laura de Magistris and colleagues,[109] Robertson did not exclude those who were already following a gluten-free diet from their analysis.

> Several studies have reported that leaky gut is present in some cases of autism and other family members

To date the de Magistris study is the most comprehensive investigation undertaken both in terms of participant numbers and the number of parameters reported on outside of simply measures of intestinal permeability. They concluded that abnormal intestinal permeability test results were present in approximately one-third of their participant group of children with autism (N = 90). They also reported that where a **gluten- and casein-free (GFCF) diet** was in place at the time of intestinal permeability testing, there was a marked change to intestinal permeability values. The effect of a GFCF diet on gut permeability in cases of autism is a theme explored by other authors[110] leading to the subsequent question of whether gut hyperpermeability might have some diagnostic value related to potential best-responders to implementation of a GFCF diet.

There is the prospect of further research to come looking at gut permeability in cases of autism. Preliminary findings have been reported from Paul Patterson and colleagues[111] extending their mouse model findings of the effects of maternal immune activation on offspring animals. Abnormal gut permeability was reported, and perhaps most excitingly, seemed to be abated to some degree by use of a specific strain of bacteria called *Bacteroides fragilis*. If replicated and applicable to humans, the implications of this work could be profound. The topic of gut bacteria, by the way, has a chapter all of its own coming up soon.

Bowel issues and autism

After all that rather long discussion on coeliac disease and leaky gut, we turn our attention back to some of the other issues related to the gut that have been talked about with autism in mind. Bowel issues generally fall into one of two categories: functional bowel problems or bowel disease. Coeliac disease falls into the latter category alongside complaints like the inflammatory bowel diseases. Symptoms like constipation and diarrhoea represent the more functional aspects of bowel disorder. As one might expect there is a link between functional bowel symptoms and bowel disease. Importantly, however, not every occasion of a problematic functional bowel habit necessarily reflects bowel disease.

Functional bowel symptoms

Alongside constipation (defined as difficulties in passing stools or incomplete defecation) and diarrhoea (the presence of loose, liquid bowel motions), symptoms such as irritable bowel syndrome (IBS) and bloating are defined as functional bowel disorders.[112] There is quite a lot of evidence to suggest that functional bowel issues might be more prevalent in certain groups of people including those who present with an **intellectual disability**.[113] Given the association between autism and intellectual disability, estimated at anywhere up to 40 per cent of cases, one could see how issues like constipation might be more readily described in this group. The precise reasons for such an over-representation of functional bowel issues are complex; it is perhaps due to dietary habits and low fibre intake for example, or reduced levels of physical activity, even as a result of side-effects following the use of certain types of medicines.

Importantly, however, this state of 'not-knowing' should not automatically lead to an assumption that such functional bowel issues are just a natural part of autism. Neither should it be used onwards as an excuse for not undertaking formal investigations when such issues are encountered to rule out known causes of such features. If we know one thing about the **ESSENCE** of autism, it is that it very rarely exists on its own in some kind of social and/or developmental vacuum.

The scientific literature examining the frequency of functional bowel problems coexisting with autism is quite consistent in its findings: functional bowel problems are not uncommon phenomena in cases of autism. Evidence following parental questioning suggest that in some cases nearly half of children with autism (46 per cent) might have a least one lifetime GI symptom.[114] This frequency reported in the Chandler study, contrasted with 22 per cent and 29 per cent reported rates for typically developing and special educational needs children in their cohort. Other reports have detailed similar differences of GI symptoms between autism and asymptomatic control populations, albeit not necessarily to the same levels of frequency.

There are obvious limitations on how functional bowel disorders are observed, examined and reported. You'll note that the words 'parental questioning' is used to determine the prevalence of bowel issues. To some, this is a double-edged sword in that yes, parents are ideally suited to talk about the bowel movements of their children, particularly if their child still requires help in toileting as a consequence of not yet achieving bowel continence and/or being under training. The down-side is that most parents might be prone to error, unless they have specifically received medical training about diagnosing bowel habits and how one distinguishes a pathological bowel habit issue from just minor difficulty in going to the toilet.

Just before anyone gets upset or irritated at our insinuation of being a non-expert, we whole-heartedly accept that parents are experts on their own children. It goes without saying that the time parents spend with their children far outweighs any other, mostly fleeting, contact by health professionals for example. But the question remains about whether a parent can be as objective as a trained external observer, particularly when it comes to determining such a medical issue.

That being said, parents of children with autism might actually be quite good at describing the bowel habits of their children. To quote from the study by Phillip Gorrindo and colleagues[115] 'parents were sensitive to the existence, although not necessarily the nature' of gastrointestinal dysfunction. In other words, when a parent says that their child might have a bowel issue, clinicians would be wise to engage in some further evaluations.

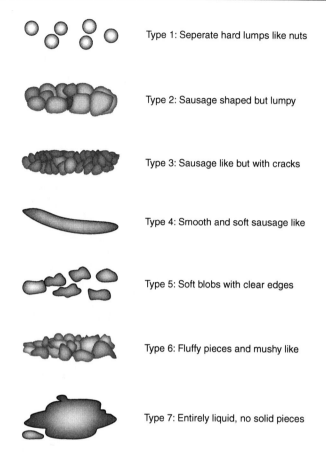

Type 1: Seperate hard lumps like nuts

Type 2: Sausage shaped but lumpy

Type 3: Sausage like but with cracks

Type 4: Smooth and soft sausage like

Type 5: Soft blobs with clear edges

Type 6: Fluffy pieces and mushy like

Type 7: Entirely liquid, no solid pieces

Figure 4.4 The Bristol Stool Chart.

Figure 4.4 shows how one of the major coding charts for stool consistency – the **Bristol Stool Chart** – categorises them.

Bowel disease

Then we have the bowel diseases and their link (or not) to autism. It's almost become an unwritten rule in some autism circles, and kingdoms, that bowel disease is not to be mentioned in the same breath as autism. We don't want to go into the politics and reasons why. Suffice to say, however, that such reluctance on the part of some areas of both medicine and research has been a significant source of distress to quite a few people.

Although there are many different types of bowel disease defined by modern medicine, it is the inflammatory bowel diseases (**IBDs**) which have taken centre-stage with autism in mind. IBD most frequently describes two conditions: ulcerative colitis (UC) and Crohn's disease. Their common denominator is inflammation of the gut. Their primary difference lies in which part of the gut is affected.

> Inflammatory bowel diseases are characterised by inflammation of the gastrointestinal (GI) tract

Several reports have detailed symptoms which seem to coincide with the descriptions of UC and/or Crohn's disease in cases of autism. That being said, there is a dearth of literature detailing how frequent such IBDs are as **comorbidity**. Kohane and colleagues[116] reported various diagnoses to be more frequently reported in cases of autism including those included under the generic heading of IBD. Their analysis based on health records suggested IBD to be over-represented, 'significantly over-represented', in those with autism, particularly in adults with autism. The absolute percentage was however small (0.83 per cent), although one should remember this was a retrospective data trawl through medical records based on received and coded diagnoses, so not necessarily covering all cases as you'll see next.

We've been careful not to just include the recognised IBDs as part of our review of the literature on autism in this area. That's because quite a few of the bowel findings being reported in cases of autism don't seem to necessarily fit snugly into one or other IBD diagnosis. Take for example the results reported by Arthur Krigsman[117] and Stephen Walker and colleagues.[118] Examined together, these reports suggested that there were some interesting features to the bowel findings reported in their respective cohorts, which might either be suggestive of 'a prodromal phase of typical inflammatory bowel disease' – that is an early stage of the condition – or perhaps more controversially, a new autism-specific variant of IBD.

There has been talk about the possibility of some cases of autism manifesting a new bowel disorder for quite a few years. The now retracted papers by Andrew Wakefield and colleagues initially proposed this suggestion, followed by various other authors

> Several reports have detailed the presence of symptoms akin to inflammatory bowel disease occurring in autism

detailing IBD-like disease as potentially being present in cases.[119] Debate continues as to the nature of the bowel observations being made, further hindered by some inconsistencies in the reports published.[120] What is clear is that irrespective of the controversy surrounding this area, further research is absolutely required and, where present, such bowel issues should be treated in the same manner as they would in the general population.

To close this rather long and quite technical chapter, but not necessarily some of the concepts we've discussed, it's worth reiterating our previous discussions about how autism (a) is not seemingly protective against developing other conditions, and (b) how some of those conditions, or indeed symptoms, might have the ability to significantly impact on day-to-day functioning for people on the autism spectrum. Our focus

> Bowel symptoms in autism deserve the same recognition and treatment as they would if present in anyone else

on the gut adds an additional dimension to the comorbidity potentially present in autism. How indeed physiology outside of merely the brain might be a good source of further experimental inquiry. We are going to talk more about the **gut–brain axis**, indeed other axes with autism in mind, but will close with reference to the paper by Micah Mazurek and colleagues[121] highlighting the potential interconnectivity of some of the symptoms we've discussed. To quote from their abstract: 'anxiety, sensory over-responsivity and GI problems are possibly interrelated phenomenon for children with **ASD**, and may have common underlying mechanisms'. We couldn't have said it better ourselves, bearing in mind the answer to the question of which causes which might not be the same for everyone.

References

83. Young E. Gut instincts: The secrets of your second brain. *New Scientist.* 2012; 2895.
84. Dodou K. and Whiteley P. Microbiomics: its growing significance in the world of medicines testing. *Pharmaceutical J.* 2013; 290: 249.
85. Sekirov I. *et al.* Gut microbiota in health and disease. *Physiol Rev.* 2010; 90: 859–904.
86. Asperger H. Psychopathology of children with celiac disease. *Ann Paediatr.* 1961; 197: 346–351
87. Fasano A. and Catassi C. Current approaches to diagnosis and treatment of celiac disease: an evolving spectrum. *Gastroenterology.* 2001; 120: 636–651.
88. Batista IC. *et al.* Autism spectrum disorder and celiac disease: no evidence for a link. *Arq Neuropsiquiatr.* 2012; 70: 28–33.
89. Barcia G. *et al.* Autism and coeliac disease. *J Autism Dev Disord.* 2008; 38: 407–408.
90. Rosenspire A. *et al.* Autism spectrum disorders are associated with an elevated autoantibody response to tissue transglutaminase-2. *Autism Res.* 2011; 4: 242–249.
91. Genuis SJ. and Bouchard TP. Celiac disease presenting as autism. *J Child Neurol.* 2010; 25: 114–119.
92. Hadjivassiliou M. *et al.* Gluten sensitivity as a neurological illness. *J Neurol Neurosurg Psychiatry* 2002; 72: 560–563.
93. Sapone A. *et al.* Spectrum of gluten-related disorders: consensus on new nomenclature and classification. *BMC Medicine* 2012; 10: 13.
94. Biesiekierski JR. *et al.* Gluten causes gastrointestinal symptoms in subjects without celiac disease: a double-blind randomized placebo-controlled trial. *Am J Gastroenterol.* 2011; 106: 508–514.
95. Sapone A. *et al.* Divergence of gut permeability and mucosal immune gene expression in two gluten associated conditions: celiac disease and gluten sensitivity. *BMC Medicine* 2011; 9: 23.
96. Wang W. *et al.* Human zonulin, a potential modulator of intestinal tight junctions. *J Cell Sci.* 2000; 113: 4435–4440.
97. Sapone A. *et al.* Zonulin upregulation is associated with increased gut permeability in subjects with type 1 diabetes and their relatives. *Diabetes.* 2006; 55: 1443–1449.
98. Fasano A. *et al.* Zonulin, a newly discovered modulator of intestinal permeability, and its expression in coeliac disease. *Lancet.* 2000; 355: 1518–1519.
99. Drago S. *et al.* Gliadin, zonulin and gut permeability: Effects on celiac and non-celiac intestinal mucosa and intestinal cell lines. *Scand J Gastroenterol.* 2006; 41: 408–419.
100. http://www.nhs.uk/conditions/leaky-gut-syndrome/Pages/Introduction.aspx (accessed June 2013).
101. Papoff P. *et al.* Gut microbial translocation in critically ill children and effects of supplementation with pre- and probiotics. *Int J Microbiol.* 2012; 2012: 151393.
102. Schneeberger EE. and Lynch RD. The tight junction: a multifunctional complex. *Am J Physiol Cell Physiol.* 2004; 286: C1213–C1228.
103. Ulluwishewa D. *et al.* Regulation of tight junction permeability by intestinal bacteria and dietary components. *J Nutr.* 2011; 141: 769–776.
104. Fasano A. Leaky gut and autoimmune diseases. *Clin Rev Allergy Immunol.* 2012; 42: 71–78.
105. Goodwin MS. *et al.* Malabsorption and cerebral dysfunction: a multivariate and comparative study of autistic children. *J Autism Child Schizophr.* 1971; 1: 48–62.
106. Goodwin MS. and Goodwin TC. In a dark mirror. *Ment Hyg.* 1969; 53: 550–563.
107. D'Eufemia P. *et al.* Abnormal intestinal permeability in children with autism. *Acta Paediatr.* 1996; 85: 1076–1079.
108. Robertson MA. *et al.* Intestinal permeability and glucagon-like peptide-2 in children with autism: a controlled pilot study. *J Autism Dev Disord.* 2008; 38: 1066–1071.
109. de Magistris L. *et al.* Alterations of the intestinal barrier in patients with autism spectrum disorders and in their first-degree relatives. *J Pediatr Gastroenterol Nutr.* 2010; 51: 418–424.

110. Whiteley P. *et al.* How could a gluten- and casein-free diet ameliorate symptoms associated with autism spectrum conditions? *Autism Insights.* 2010; 2: 39–53.

111. Hughes V. Blog post: *Probiotic curbs autism features in mouse model.* 2012. http://sfari.org/news-and-opinion/conference-news/2012/society-for-neuroscience-2012/probiotic-curbs-autism-features-in-mouse-model.

112. Longstreth GF. *et al.* Functional bowel disorders. *Gastroenterology.* 2006; 130: 1480–1491.

113. Böhmer CJ. *et al.* The prevalence of constipation in institutionalized people with intellectual disability. *J Intellect Disabil Res.* 2001; 45: 212–218.

114. Chandler S. *et al.* Parent-reported gastro-intestinal symptoms in children with autism spectrum disorders. *J Autism Dev Disord.* February 2013.

115. Gorrindo P. *et al.* Gastrointestinal dysfunction in autism: parental report, clinical evaluation, and associated factors. *Autism Res.* 2012; 5: 101–108.

116. Kohane IS. *et al.* The co-morbidity burden of children and young adults with autism spectrum disorders. *PLoS One.* 2012; 7: e33224.

117. Krigsman A. *et al.* Clinical presentation and histologic findings at ileocolonoscopy in children with autistic spectrum disorder and chronic gastrointestinal symptoms. *Autism Insights.* 2010; 2: 11.

118. Walker SJ. *et al.* Identification of unique gene expression profile in children with regressive autism spectrum disorder (ASD) and ileocolitis. *PLoS ONE.* 2013; 8: e58058.

119. Balzola F. *et al.* Panenteric IBD-like disease in a patient with regressive autism shown for the first time by the wireless capsule enteroscopy: another piece in the jigsaw of this gut-brain syndrome? *Am J Gastroenterol.* 2005; 100: 979–981.

120. Chen B. *et al.* Abnormal gastrointestinal histopathology in children with autism spectrum disorders. *J Pediatr Gastroenterol Nutr.* February 2011.

121. Mazurek MO. *et al.* Anxiety, sensory over-responsivity, and gastrointestinal problems in children with autism spectrum disorders. *J Abnorm Child Psychol.* 2013; 41: 165–176.

RECIPES

Flaxseed porridge

We will warn you that this recipe does have a strange 'gloopy' texture which might not be to everyone's taste. But if you do enjoy it, it's full of nutrition and warms you up.

Ingredients per person

30 grams of flaxseed
2 teaspoons of peanut butter
2 teaspoons of cocoa powder
½ teaspoon of cinnamon
¼ teaspoon of pure stevia or a sweetener or sugar as you prefer
60 millilitres of water

Method

Mix all the dry ingredients and the peanut butter in a cereal bowl, add 60mls of boiling water, mix well and leave for 2 minutes to let the flaxseed absorb the water. You might need to add a little more water to reach a consistency you prefer.

Sprinkling of nutritional science

There is quite a scientific reputation behind those little seeds derived from the flax plant. As well as being a great source of dietary fibre essential for 'keeping us regular', flaxseeds are a good source of omega-3 fatty acids (alpha-linolenic acid, ALA), normally found in oily fish. Omega-3 fatty acids have been linked to everything from good heart health to good cognitive health and indeed improvements in some of the symptoms of autism and conditions such as attention-deficit hyperactivity disorder (**ADHD**). Added to the oestrogen-like chemicals, lignans, also present in flaxseed, as being a good antioxidant, these tiny seeds pack quite a health punch.

Hot or cold cereal mix

A cereal that's versatile to your morning mood.

Ingredients

220 grams rolled oats (check to ensure that they gluten-free)
115 grams of raisins
50 grams of chopped flaked almonds
35 grams of dried shredded coconut
30 grams of ground flaxseed
50 grams of pumpkin seeds
¼ teaspoon of cinnamon
¼ teaspoon of salt

Method

Combine all the ingredients in a large bowl and mix well. Store in an airtight container until ready to eat. To prepare hot: in a small bowl, combine equal parts hot water and oatmeal mix (for example, 1 cup water, 1 cup oatmeal), stir, and cover. Leave to sit for about 3 minutes and enjoy. Or served cold, you can soak it with apple juice the night before or serve with dairy-free milk of your choice

Sprinkling of nutritional science

Although the topic of continued speculation on whether oats are in fact free of gluten as a result of contamination with other gluten-containing grains, in cases of **coeliac disease** – an exquisite sensitivity to gluten – oats are not generally thought to be toxic. As well as being a great source of magnesium, much of the reported health benefits linked to oat consumption stem from their soluble fibre content (beta-glucan) and the link between oat consumption and lower levels of LDL (so-called bad) **cholesterol**.

Avocado fudgesicles

Unusual ingredients which create an amazing fudgy, sweet iced treat (makes 4–8 lollies).

Ingredients

8 tinned prunes with stones removed
125 millilitres/½ cup of apple juice that prunes are tinned in
1 large avocado, pitted
85 grams/¼ cup of honey
3 tablespoons of cocoa powder
2 teaspoons of vanilla
A pinch sea salt

Method

Place the prunes into your blender or processor and add ½ cup apple juice. Add in the remaining ingredients and blend until very smooth and creamy. Depending on your blender, you may need to add a little extra water. Pour into small bowls and serve as pudding or pour into lollipop moulds and freeze for at least 6 hours. Run under hot water to release.

Sprinkling of nutritional science

Not one of the most visually appetising of foods, prunes are an under-consumed food which can transform many dishes. Most people will think of the proposed laxative effect of prunes which in part stems from their high phenolic content. Prunes, however, provide so much more than 'keeping someone regular' because of the high level of antioxidants they contain. A good source of potassium potentially important for good heart health, and of boron, optimal levels of which are linked to a reduced risk of osteoporosis, prunes aren't necessarily all about the toilet.

Lettuce wraps

A great tortilla substitute inspired from the USA, this bright and colourful recipe is ideal for a family picnic (serves 4).

Ingredients

For the refried beans
2 tablespoons of oil (olive or rapeseed)
100 grams bacon, finely chopped
1 medium onion, finely chopped
Black pepper
1 (250 g) tin of beans (cannellini, pinto or black beans), drained and rinsed

A selection of large lettuce leaves
½ red pepper
½ avocado
1 tablespoon of lime juice
½ red chili, finely chopped (optional)

Method

Add 1 tablespoon of oil to a pan and lightly fry the bacon. Set the bacon aside, add the rest of the oil and the onion and cook gently until they are soft and translucent. If you want a chunky mixture mash the beans with something like a potato masher or for a finer texture add to a food processor or blender until you have the beans as fine as you like. Mix or blend in the onions, bacon and black pepper. Wash the lettuce leaves and down one side of the leaf put a line of refried beans, red pepper, chili and sliced avocado drizzled with lime. Then tuck in one end of the lettuce and roll.

Sprinkling of nutritional science

Avocados are fruit powerhouses packed with **vitamins**, **minerals** and monounsaturated fatty acids. Extracts from avocados have been experimentally studied with lots of potential applications in mind including properties linked to the lowering of cholesterol for those with elevated cholesterol levels. Their use in various skin preparations pays homage to their role in supporting healthy-looking skin and even as a potential therapy for skin conditions including psoriasis.

Tuscan bean stew

A warm filling stew perfect for an autumn or winter night (serves 4).

Ingredients

1 tablespoon of olive oil
50 g pancetta
1 red onion
1 stick of celery, finely diced
1 small carrot, peeled and finely diced

1 teaspoon of thyme
4 garlic cloves, crushed
1 tablespoon of tomato purée
2 bay leaves
1 tin of tomatoes
1 small tin of cannellini beans
1 small tin of kidney beans
1 baby courgette or half a medium courgette, finely diced
Half a red pepper, de-seeded and finely diced
1 sweet potato, peeled and diced
250 millilitres of vegetable stock
1 teaspoon of honey
1 teaspoon of black pepper

Method

Put a large heavy-based pan on the heat and add the olive oil. Chop the onions finely and add to the pan with the pancetta and allow to cook slowly for a few minutes. Add the celery, carrot and thyme and allow to sweat for 2–3 minutes. Add the garlic and tomato purée and cook for a further few minutes, then add the rest of the ingredients and allow to simmer gently for 40 minutes

Sprinkling of nutritional science

Whilst the question of whether celery is truly a negative calorie food – consuming it burns more calories than it contains – continues to be discussed, there are several other reasons why celery should be included as part of a nutritionally balanced diet. Celery contains various chemicals thought to be active against various conditions including high blood pressure.

Rice stuffing

Make a batch of this stuffing to serve with pork (serves 4).

Ingredients

1 onion, peeled and finely chopped
½ tablespoon of oil (olive or rapeseed)
4 tablespoons of cooked rice
6 dried prunes or apricots
1 grated apple
1 dessertspoon of toasted flaked almonds
½ lemon zest only
1 egg
1 teaspoon of herbs such as thyme and/or sage

Method

Heat the oil in a pan and gently sweat the onion until it is tender for about 5 minutes. Place the onion in a bowl and mix together with the rest of the ingredients. This stuffing can be placed in an ovenproof greased dish and baked for 25 minutes or it can be placed on top of a cut of meat (e.g. pork chop) or used as a stuffing for chicken (cooking times will vary according to the meat selected).

Sprinkling of nutritional science

'An apple a day keeps the doctor away.' So went the proverb, and the facts about apples seem to reinforce their health-giving status. Consumption of both the flesh and skin of apples has been linked to the relief of various conditions via compounds such as quercetin and ursolic acid.

Chapter 5

The gut microbiome

We're at war. In these modern days of **antibiotics** and other antibacterial products used to sanitise ourselves and the world around us, bacteria have unfortunately taken on the title of aggressor in many quarters. If we mention the name *E. coli* what's the first thing that pops into your mind? A relatively harmless family of 'bugs' which live in our **gut**, or all those news stories of food poisoning and media headlines of 'flesh-eating bacteria'? It's little wonder that the words 'kills 99.9% of all bacteria' are readily found throughout the modern home.

We're not saying that bacteria, certain types of bacteria present under certain conditions and circumstances, are not associated with ill-health and even early mortality. But the word 'bacteria' represents one of the most abundant life forms on the planet: diverse in nature and presentation. To say all bacteria are bad and disease-causing is an over-reaction. And you should know from our discussions so far that we're not overly keen on generalisation.

Microbiomics – the science of bacteria – has already received mention in the previous chapter. You might be wondering why we just don't say bacteriology or something similar to describe the study of bacteria instead of calling it an –omic. Well, quite a few of our sciences are tending more and more to use the term –omic in their title to denote 'study' and 'collectivity'; think back also to **epigenomics** and the science of the epigenome. One might argue it's just a trendy rebrand. Like it or not, however, we are living in the age of the –omic and its 'big data' implications.

> Microbiomics is the study of bacteria and their effects

Bacteria have been studied for quite a while. Louis Pasteur (1822–1895) is credited as being an early pioneer of the study of bacteria. His studies supported even earlier suggestions of a germ theory of disease – microorganisms causing infection – and were fundamental to our modern-day understanding of bacteria as being potential agents of disease. That Pasteur also invented the process of pasteurisation – heating and rapidly cooling a food to inhibit bacterial growth – is testament to his continued influence today.

Most people will probably have heard of another important name on the early microbiomics scene: Sir Alexander Fleming (1881–1955). Fleming shared the Nobel Prize for his discovery of the mould which was eventually turned into penicillin, one of the world's first mass-produced antibiotics. His discovery is subsequently credited with saving the lives of millions of people who might otherwise have succumbed to what are now seen as trivial conditions and infections following the introduction of antibiotics.

The intervening years have seen many important developments in our understanding of bacteria. One milestone in bacteria research was the publication of first results[122] from the Human Microbiome Project (HMP) in 2012. Realising that humans like other animals are teaming with bacteria, the HMP set out to map the various types of bacteria that colonise us and call us home, to build up a detailed picture of which bacteria are where and in what quantity. The sheer volume of data generated from this project hinted that there is certainly variation among the types of bacteria which inhabit us according to different regions of the body. Importantly also, was the realisation that there are significant interactions between our body as host and bacteria as our passengers which may very well impact on our health and wellbeing.

Our bacterial masters

It's been estimated that an adult human carries over a kilogram of bacteria in their gut. Spread throughout the gut, bacteria have traditionally been thought of as merely aiding digestion of our food and perhaps producing some amount of various nutrients, such as one form of **vitamin B12,** for example.[123] The notion that the bacteria which reside in our gut – the second brain – may actually impact on our 'first brain' functions was a difficult concept to swallow.

In recent times however, evidence has begun to emerge suggestive that our gut microbiome may very well be extending its reach into areas well beyond the GI tract. Rodent studies looking at the impact of the presence or absence of gut bacteria on observed behaviours have reported differences in relation to anxiety-like behaviours for example.[124] Just as important is the possibility that behaviour may influence gut bacteria[125] suggesting a dynamic bi-directional relationship between the two. There's even a suggestion that gut bacteria may be 'essential' for the achievement of specific developmental milestones such as social behaviours[126] at least in mice. Psychobacteriomics is a word that springs to mind to draw attention to the psychology–bacteria and bacteria–psychology links being proposed.

The observant reader has probably spotted the potential flaw in the research we've highlighted as supportive of gut bacteria and behaviour being a dynamic exchange. Rodents such as mice and rats are not human beings. As much as we think that such animal behaviour might overlap with human behaviour, it doesn't. Indeed it can never truly mimic the complexity of humans and the unique and multiple interactions we have with our environment.

That's not to say, however, that humans, and human behaviour, have not been looked at with gut bacteria in mind. Take for example the study by Rao and colleagues[127] looking at the effect of alterations to the gut bacteria following supplementation with a **probiotic** – bacteria thought to carry some health benefit – in cases of **chronic fatigue syndrome (CFS)**. Their controlled study suggested that those in receipt of the probiotic showed changes to their gut bacteria profile corresponding also with indications of a decrease in reported anxiety-related symptoms when compared to a placebo (a dummy or inert treatment). Likewise the results reported by Kirsten Tillisch and colleagues[128] detailing alterations to brain activity as shown by **functional magnetic resonance imaging (fMRI)** following supplementation with a probiotic are fascinating. Interestingly they detected changes in connectivity of parts of the brain in areas related to emotion and sensory processing.

The precise mechanisms of effect accounting for these examples of gut bacteria influencing aspects of human behaviour and even brain functions are still

Gut bacteria have been suggested to be able to influence behaviour the source of some speculation. As we saw in our previous discussions on the ability of certain gut bacteria to make vitamins and other nutrients, it is conceivable that changes to the gut microbiome might similarly be influencing the production of other compounds and chemicals of relevance to mood and other facets of behaviour. One might equally argue for some important role for the **vagus nerve** – the 'hotline' link between the gut and brain – as being active in this process.[129] Perhaps more speculative is the potential effect that such bacterial changes may be having on processes like the **leaky gut** and, onwards, any implications for immune system changes which might result. Immune function and its wider role outside of fighting infections will be discussed later.

Autism and the gut microbiome

What we hope we've illustrated so far in our introductory discussions about the gut microbiome is that (a) the study of gut bacteria is still in its infancy, (b) gut bacteria might however be doing so much more than just helping to digest food and (c) gut bacteria might be an integral part of the so-called **gut–brain axis**. With all that in mind, we're going to look at some of the research undertaken examining the gut microbiome in relation to cases of autism. Some readers may find some of this information a little heavy going to begin with but stick with it, because this area may well turn out to represent something really important to conditions like autism.

As one might expect, the possibility that gut bacteria may show some involvement with the presentation of the autisms is still a relatively recent hypothesis. Interestingly, like many areas of the autism research landscape, it was a parent of a child with autism who seems to have the honour of first raising the possibility of a link between elements of the gut microbiome and autism in the scientific literature.[130] Although her ideas were speculative at the time of publication in 1998, Ellen Bolte, the mother of a man with autism, posited a link between several elements – early antibiotic use disrupting gut flora, the onset of autism, colonisation of the gut with neurotoxin-producing bacteria, gastrointestinal symptoms – as potentially being linked. Her report was rooted in her own experiences of her son's seemingly typical development and subsequent regression into autism.

For those who have followed the winding autism research path down the years, it should be no surprise that a parent of a child with autism might have been the first to ask such a question. Autism research is positively filled with parents with children with autism making often important discoveries, whether based on their own experiences or driven into autism research as a function of their child's diagnosis, complementary to the variety of other endeavours that parents (and grandparents) have been instrumental in setting up.

> Various studies have reported differences in the types of gut bacteria present in cases of autism

Going back to the gut microbiome and autism suggestion, the name Ellen Bolte has also subsequently appeared on other, very much more experiment-based, papers.[131,132] We'll attend shortly to the Sandler paper[131] looking at what happened following the use of a quite powerful antibiotic to alter the gut flora in cases of autism. The paper by Feingold and colleagues[132] represented one of the first attempts to characterise the gut microbiota in cases of autism compared with control stool samples. They reported increased levels of clostridial species – a bacterial class of the Firmicutes – to be present in stool samples from their small cohort of children with autism compared with controls. They also identified several bacterial differences in tissue samples derived from various parts of the gut in their late-onset autism group. The reward for Bolte's contribution to this rising star of autism research areas was to have her name immortalised on one of the species isolated in later studies[133] – *Clostridium bolteae*.

Various other studies have reached similar conclusions as to the research we've already highlighted, albeit focused on other species of bacteria given the wide diversity seemingly present in the gut. Clostridia is however a word mentioned quite consistently.[134]

We're going to draw your attention to two other types of gut bacteria potentially linked to cases of autism. Originally identified in the faeces of dogs, levels of the genus *Sutterella* were initially thought to show linkage to Crohn's disease following some small-scale analysis of human stool samples. Subsequent investigations have questioned this proposed link[135] and on more than one occasion.[136] With autism in mind, the results reported by Brent Williams and colleagues[137] suggested some potential role for this rod bacteria which thrives under low-oxygen and anaerobic (lacking oxygen) conditions. You'll hear more about the research of Brent Williams in later discussions but in this trial it was a case of identifying *Sutterella* in various tissue samples taken from the gut of children with autism and control participants. Perhaps importantly, the children with autism included for study were all presenting with GI issues. Williams reported finding evidence of *Sutterella* gene sequences in over half of his group compared with none of his much smaller control group. Immune responses to *Sutterella* were also detected in some of the children with autism, potentially indicative of bacterial translocation and speculatively, potential issues with gut permeability (leaky gut). Subsequent work has similarly reported a possible connection between autism and *Sutterella*[138]. That being said, the relevance of elevated numbers of *Sutterella* bacteria to the onset or pathology of autism is currently unknown.

> Bacteria belonging to the genus *Sutterella* have been reported in cases of autism

Having made referenced the work of Dr Manya Angley and colleagues in replicating some of the initial findings with *Sutterella* in mind, we turn also to other bacterial research published by her team in relation to autism. Lynn Wang published an interesting paper[139] reporting lower levels of bacteria called *Akkermansia muciniphila* (pronounced Akker-man-sia), described as **mucolytic** bacteria – involved in making mucus less thick and sticky. The authors speculated that lower levels of *A. muciniphila* in their autism cohort might be indicative of 'mucus barrier changes', as in similar findings in cases of **IBD**.[140] This again, brings us back to the gut permeability issues previously discussed with autism in mind.

Outside of the gut barrier speculation, *A. muciniphila* has also provoked interest in relation to a more general health-related issue, obesity.[141] The suggestion of a link between obesity and lower levels of the bacteria (at least in mice), together with some very beneficial effects on some of the presentations of **metabolic syndrome,** received quite a lot of interest. Whilst replication in human beings is still required, one has to wonder whether the presence of lower levels of *A. muciniphila* in cases of autism might also represent similar risk of obesity[74] rather than any autism-specific connection. Or maybe even shared gut permeability issues being present in both obesity and autism?[142] Just speculating, sorry.

On the basis of the collective work we've presented looking at levels and species of gut bacteria either derived from stools or biopsy samples, it might look at though gut bacteria is absolutely implicated in autism. Like seemingly everything related to autism, however, nothing is so

> Siblings of people with autism may also show similar gut bacteria profiles

simple. Take for example the paper by Gondalia and colleagues[143] reporting no significant differences in gut bacteria between children with autism and their asymptomatic siblings. Whilst one could argue that use of a sibling group as the only control group is perhaps not the ideal scenario (same food, same drink, same environment) the study nevertheless highlights the fact that the relationship with gut bacteria, if they are involved in cases of autism, is not necessarily going to be straightforward.

Bacterial metabolites in urine

Whilst the inspection of stool and gut biopsy samples represent a very good way of looking at what bacteria are present in our deepest, darkest bowels, it's not the only way. Taking the example from the Brent Williams paper,[137] if you assume that bacterial translocation might be an issue, you could check blood samples for antibodies – the immune system reacting to a foreign invader like bacteria or a virus – generated against a specific type of bacteria. There's also the possibility of looking in other less invasive ways at biological fluids such as urine[144] based on the knowledge that gut bacteria can produce their own suite of chemicals and compounds, as with the vitamin B12 example[123] we discussed previously.

Indeed, urine has been a focus for quite a lot of study with autism in mind. Sometimes, often coincidentally, investigations have isolated compounds to be present and potentially of gut bacterial origins. Before heading through some of the key findings in this area, it might be useful for us to pass comment on the various ways and means that research analyses, detects and classifies compounds detected in fluids like urine.

Although you might not be aware of it, from an analytical point of view, urine is precious stuff. OK, we know that it's a waste product and generally speaking not something that people necessarily want think about as being a data-rich resource. But all manner of conditions have been, and continue to be, looked at based on the analysis of urine and the science of something called **metabolomics**.

We don't necessarily want to provide a detailed overview of metabolomics (yet another of those –omics) and what it is and does. Suffice to say that it involves screening urine or other types of biological samples based on some very technical and precise equipment and then applying some very complicated statistical models to the often huge amounts of data on the small molecules (metabolites) collected to, hopefully, identify which compounds are present and importantly which are relevant to the condition or disease being looked at.[145]

Early reports of urine compounds derived or modified by gut bacteria being found in cases of autism, whilst interesting, might also require some degree of caution. Take for example the findings reported by Lis and colleagues.[146] Their reports of various 'abnormalities' in the urinary excretions noted in their cohort of children with autism have to some extent been replicated in later work. Their methods, however, based on the gold standard at the time of publication (1976) are by today's standards simple and not entirely conducive to accurate determination of specific compounds. Indeed, one of the authors of this book has similarly reported results based on such imprecise methods[147] (we'll be mentioning the letters '**IAG**' in relation to autism in a subsequent chapter).

More recent work utilising technologies with fancy names like **mass spectrometry (MS)** and nuclear magnetic resonance (NMR) provides an altogether more accurate overview of what urinary compounds are potentially important to autism and their relative abundance compared to controls. The results reported by Yap and colleagues[148] are credited with heralding an important point in the application of metabolomics to autism. Including a familiar name in the authorship group (Manya Angley) and also one of the big names in the science of metabolomics, Jeremy Nicholson, their results were broadly supportive of some of the earlier findings from Lis and colleagues: 'a perturbation in the tryptophan-nicotinic acid metabolic pathway'. **Tryptophan**, by the way, is an **amino acid** similar to the units of those strings of pearls we talked about when describing **coeliac disease**. It's also the starting material for some important compounds such as **serotonin** (that neurotransmitter) and melatonin, a compound which some readers might have heard about with regards to its link to the sleep-wake cycle.

> Various chemicals derived from bacteria have been detected in urine samples from people with autism

Other research groups have also reported on the detection of urinary compounds whose origins can be traced back to the action of gut bacteria[149,150] on things like amino acids. It is perhaps no coincidence that, in particular, the focus has been on a specific class of amino acids, the aromatic amino acids such as tryptophan, tyrosine and phenylalanine, as potentially being differentially modified by certain gut bacteria. Although the details are beyond the scope of this book, any readers interested in finding out more about how bacteria can modify these amino acids potentially with autism in mind would be advised the read the excellent paper by Andrew Clayton.[151]

Once again, we're not trying to promote a position whereby metabolites in urine or other biological fluids are going to somehow yield an 'autism compound' universal to everyone with autism. If specific gut bacteria play a role in generating specific compounds or metabolites, the identification of such bacteria by proxy (urine analysis) is the goal of such research in addition to other methods. Importantly, one has to realise that this is to some degree quite a dynamic process influenced by various factors including dietary intake and the use of various medicines. In short, it's complicated.

Antibiotics and autism: a therapeutic option?

There is no doubt that **antibiotics** – medicines used to kill or inhibit the growth of bacteria – are lifesavers. One might even argue that they are one of the key advances in the history of medicine given the numbers of people who owe their lives to antibiotics. But as with many advances that we seemingly make against the multitude of agents that would debilitate us or even kill us, these 'bugs' have also developed the tools to survive.

In the case of bacteria, two of the main tools in their arsenal are their sheer numbers and their striking ability to adapt. Compared with the slow pace of evolutionary adaptation that humans possess, bacteria are vastly superior and able to pass on resistance to specific antibiotics as a consequence of their natural selection. Their numbers mean that what might take thousands of years for humans, can be done in a matter of years in bacteria. And they're starting to fight back as shown, for instance, by the example of methicillin-resistant *Staphylococcus aureus* (MRSA) which is worrying quite a few very eminent people.

The other important thing to note about antibiotics is that they are generally not very selective about where and which bacteria they target. That's not to say that there is just one antibiotic which will target all the different types of bacteria; that's the reason medicine has a range of different antibiotics. But when you swallow an antibiotic to treat a bacterial infection, it is, as science writer Carl Zimmer described[152] something akin to swallowing 'a grenade' in terms of the potential effects on the gut microbiota as a whole.

The idea being that even if certain pathogenic – disease-causing – bacteria are destroyed during the antibiotic onslaught, it's more than likely that some 'friendlies' will also suffer the same fate. Such disruption then alters the balance of the various types of bacteria present in the gut described as a state of **dysbiosis** and, in extreme cases, bacteria such as *Clostridium difficile* can become established, with onward effects.

If it all sounds a little bit unbelievable, readers would be well advised to read the report by Goldenberg and colleagues[153] on the possible requirements for probiotic supplementation to prevent any functional bowel disorders as a consequence of antibiotic-induced *C. diff.* infection. We might also throw into the conversation the suggestion that early antibiotic use might even be related to an elevated risk for more chronic bowel problems such as the inflammatory bowel diseases.[154] Such is the growing relationship between our gut flora and our bowel habits and health.

Before, however, we enter any debates on medicine being thrown back to the nineteenth century as a result of widespread antibiotic resistance, we'd like to discuss some of the interest in antibiotics in relation to autism. As well as describing the contribution of Ellen Bolte to autism research, we made mention of the paper by Richard Sandler and colleagues.[131] Their results suggested that following administration of quite a powerful antibiotic, vancomycin – in some quarters talked about as the antibiotic of last resort because of its use when other antibiotics have failed – to children with regressive-onset autism, there were some notable changes observed in quite a few of their small participant group (8/10). Bearing in mind the methodology adopted based solely on behavioural observation and the use of a non-blinded case study design, their results hinted that if early disruption to the gut microflora was present among some cases of autism for whatever reason, there may be pharmacological means to intervene and 'reset' any gut bacteria dysbiosis.

It would be easy to speculate that the reported effects of vancomycin were centrally due to it targeting bacteria like *C. diff.* given its more usual applications against gram-positive bacteria (all to do with its colour of staining and cell wall constitution). Even easier when one takes into account the related comment by Linday[155] on the potential usefulness of a yeast called *Saccharomyces boulardii* for cases of autism and functional GI symptoms, given the actions of *S. boulardii* on *C. diff.* infection.[156] But alas, confirmatory evidence supporting these initial reports is sadly lacking at the current time. The associated report of the effect of vancomycin being only short-term might also hint that there is some degree of bacterial self-correction at work such that episodic changes to gut bacteria are unlikely to bring about sustained changes to behavioural presentation. Certainly, long-term use of vancomycin is not generally a suitable strategy.

Given research looking at other antibiotics as potential intervention tools for autism or conditions manifesting autistic symptoms, one might also speculate that any effect is not necessarily exclusively due to an action on gut bacteria. Take for example some of the collected work looking at the antibiotic D-cycloserine as a possible therapeutic option for cases of autism[157] or even more tentatively, minocycline,[158] the insinuation being that there may be more central effects also being observed on, for instance, specific biological receptors such as N-methyl D-aspartate (NMDA).[159] One might even speculate on their action against other organisms such as **parasites** bearing in mind the current evidence base on specific organisms.[160] Trials of such antibiotics for other use with other conditions such as **schizophrenia** similarly hint at extra-intestinal effects.[161]

> Antibiotics used to kill certain bacteria have been suggested as an intervention for autism

Antibiotics and autism: the other side of the sword

Whilst antibiotics may potentially offer clues and an intervention option for some cases of the autisms, whether in relation to core symptoms or by more peripheral means, not everyone might be so inclined to sing their praises. Again we draw on the experiences described by Ellen Bolte of her son's regression into autism coincidental to his receipt of multiple courses of antibiotics to treat recurrent ear infection. The suggestion is that antibiotic use may be a double-edged sword when it comes to autism.

The correlations suggested between early ear infections treated by multiple courses of antibiotics being linked to the onset of autism have been explored in both the lay and the scientific literature. Outside of the speculative 'what if' reports, it does appear that ear infections may be more frequent in children with autism.[162] Indeed there have also been case reports linking the course of such infections with the presentation of symptoms.[163] Similarly, there is some evidence that children with autism presenting with ear infections may also be more likely to use more antibiotics than asymptomatic children.[164]

Of course these correlations do not prove causation. It is possible that those children who are destined to develop autism might be more prone to ear infections as a result of physiological or structural differences in ear anatomy. Said anatomy might be a feature of their autism presentation and the accompanying use of antibiotics is merely a distracting factor. On the other hand though, knowing how antibiotics can and do affect things like gut bacteria, perhaps even altering risk of conditions like the IBDs, and onwards that whole 'gut bacteria might influence behaviour' hypothesis, one cannot discount a potential effect, even if only an ancillary one.

Probiotics (and prebiotics)

Outside of the attempts at blanket eradication of gut bacteria for whatever purpose, another strategy has seemingly engulfed our modern-day lives based on the theory of competition: probiotics. We've already talked about the Rao study[127] utilising a probiotic to alter one particular aspect of CFS. Such probiotics are suggested to work on the balance of various bacteria which are present in the gut and assume that the introduction of more beneficial species of bacteria might reduce both the numbers and effects of less beneficial species. Indeed most people have something like a probiotic in their fridge or larder. Probiotics are normally included as part of those yoghurts or yoghurt drinks, and the perceived benefits from such preparations have dazzled an increasingly health-conscious consumer.

Whether probiotics are actually one of the so-called 'superfoods' or merely a fad based on clever marketing probably depends on your viewpoint. Certainly there is evidence that some probiotic products may very well impact on the experience of conditions like IBS[165] among other things. Drawing on the connection between functional bowel issues and certain types of bacteria like *C. diff.* one might expect such a link to be made. But the question of whether we can fundamentally alter and sustain such changes to the organisation of our gut bacteria, the same bacteria with which the body grows up and the immune system becomes so friendly, as a result of probiotic supplementation still remains unanswered.

The current literature looking at autism and probiotic use is still quite limited. Critchfield and colleagues[166] provided a useful overview of the rationale and evidence for at least entertaining the possibility that specific probiotic preparations might be something to look at with autism in mind. Complementary to the suggestion that certain probiotic bacterial strains might have some interesting effects on gut permeability in mouse models of autism[111] and some very preliminary data looking at GI function as a consequence of supplementation,[167] the door is still open for further investigations being done.

Of perhaps equal or greater importance to gut bacteria and the emphasis of this book being on food is the concept of prebiotics. As their name suggests, prebiotics are concerned with foods or other entities which are able to stimulate the growth of certain bacteria in the gut which convey a potential health benefit. The food of our good gut bacteria you might say. Still a relatively new

> Probiotics to promote 'good' bacteria have been suggested as an intervention for autism

concept when it comes to food science, there is still some controversy over what is and isn't a prebiotic. Generally speaking things like non-digestible **carbohydrates** (oligosaccharides) are prebiotics (we'll be coming on to carbohydrates quite soon). We've mentioned how some foods are a great source of prebiotics. Indeed quite a few of them are GFCF, including chicory, artichoke, garlic and leeks. As the literature on probiotics indicates, there is still more to be done on prebiotics and autism from a research point of view.

Yuck factor 10

We've covered antibiotics and probiotics as the primary ways suggested and being used to try and effect change to the gut microbiome in autism and other conditions. You'd probably think that would be just about everything that could be done. But what happens if we were to suggest that there were another possibility which might accomplish such a task? An approach probably not meant for the faint-hearted. Welcome to the world of the faecal bacteriotherapy, also known as the faecal transplant or **faecal microbiota transplant (FMT)**.

As the various names suggest, the basics of FMT involve a donation. A donation based on the stools of a donor being blended into a form more ready for 'insertion' into another person, often via a nasogastric tube, hopefully to be followed by a fundamental shift in the gut microbiota and some improvement in health. Whilst not necessarily sounding all that appealing, there is some good evidence emerging to suggest that FMT might have an important role to play in conditions like *C. diff.* infection, for example.[168] Indeed so much so that there was some chatter that the US Food & Drug Administration (FDA) might start to legislate on how and under what circumstances FMT might be used.

Probably one of the more well-known names attached to FMT is that of Dr Thomas Borody. Perhaps more famous for his role in the development of triple therapy[169] for the eradication of the bacterium *Helicobacter pylori*, and its relationship with peptic ulcers, Borody has speculated on the potential many and varied uses of FMT in relation to conditions as diverse as the IBDs to autoimmune conditions even possibly with neurodevelopmental disorders in mind.[170] Chronic fatigue syndrome (CFS) has also been mentioned.

Before anyone gets the wrong impression of our inclusion of FMT in our discussions, we are not suggesting that FMT could or should be indicated for autism. Unless, that is, the person is suffering from a C. diff. infection; this, as is clear from our previous chapters, is not outside the realms of possibility given that autism is seemingly protective of nothing when it comes to **comorbidity**, and given that such an infection is recurrent, as most studies show. Added to the fact that we still know comparatively little as to what part of the transplant is active against infection, which potential safety issues need to be considered[171] and whether donor characteristics might be important at the time of donation, there's still much to do on FMT.

Rethinking bacteria

After reading this chapter some readers might be wondering if this is actually a book about autism. To entertain the idea that the autisms might not necessarily be an exclusively brain-based condition / state / disability calls for quite a major rethink. Yes, people might have heard other discussions about autism being a whole body condition, but the suggestion that something like the gut microbiome might so overtly affect either risk of autism or overt presentation of behavioural signs and symptoms is quite difficult to comprehend.

You're right to say that the research base in this area still has some significant gaps. That and some of the suggestions said to affect gut bacteria not necessarily being particularly attractive therapeutic options, particularly where important decisions on things like safety and side-effects, both short- and long-term, need to be weighed up against possible advantages.

But autism is not the only condition diagnosed solely on the basis of presented behaviour facing the question of whether the gut microbiome might be playing some role. The chicken-or-egg question of depression and C. diff. infection has been discussed by some groups.[172] Depression as a comorbidity in some cases of autism is an 'add-on' which we have not made mention of in our previous chapters. Similarly we have not discussed the potentially modifying role of conditions like **stomach** acidity in relation to autism – in particular, hypochlorhydria or low gastric acid production[132] – given some interesting speculations around 'the sieve hypothesis' on how stomach acidity is quite a good bacteriocide.[173] Once again, it's complicated.

> Our relationship with our gut bacteria is a complicated one which we're only just starting to probe

References

122. The Human Microbiome Project Consortium. A framework for human microbiome research. *Nature.* 2012; 486: 215–221.
123. Albert MJ. *et al.* Vitamin B12 synthesis by human small intestinal bacteria. *Nature.* 1980; 283: 781–782.
124. Neufeld KM. *et al.* Reduced anxiety-like behavior and central neurochemical change in germ-free mice. *Neurogastroenterol Motil.* 2011; 23: 255–264.
125. Bailey MT. *et al.* Exposure to a social stressor alters the structure of the intestinal microbiota: implications for stressor-induced immunomodulation. *Brain Behav Immun.* 2011; 25: 397–407.
126. Desbonnet L. *et al.* Microbiota is essential for social development in the mouse. *Mol Psychiatr.* May 2013.
127. Rao AV. *et al.* A randomized, double-blind, placebo-controlled pilot study of a probiotic in emotional symptoms of chronic fatigue syndrome. *Gut Pathog.* 2009; 1: 6.
128. Tillisch K. *et al.* Consumption of fermented milk product with probiotic modulates brain activity. *Gastroenterology.* 2013; 144: 1394–1401.
129. Forsythe P. *et al.* On communication between gut microbes and the brain. *Curr Opin Gastroenterol.* 2012; 28: 557–562.

130. Bolte ER. Autism and *Clostridium tetani*. *Med Hypotheses*. 1998; 51: 133–144.

131. Sandler RH. *et al*. Short-term benefit from oral vancomycin treatment of regressive-onset autism. *J Child Neurol*. 2000; 15: 429–435.

132. Feingold SM. *et al*. Gastrointestinal microflora studies in late-onset autism. *Clin Infect Dis*. 2002; 35: S6–S16.

133. Song Y. *et al*. *Clostridium bolteae* sp. nov., isolated from human sources. *Syst Appl Microbiol*. 2003; 26: 84–89.

134. Parracho HM. *et al*. Differences between the gut microflora of children with autistic spectrum disorders and that of healthy children. *J Med Microbiol*. 2005; 54: 987–991.

135. Mukhopadhya I. *et al*. A comprehensive evaluation of colonic mucosal isolates of *Sutterella wadsworthensis* from inflammatory bowel disease. *PLoS One*. 2011; 6: e27076.

136. Hansen R. *et al*. The microaerophilic microbiota of de-novo paediatric inflammatory bowel disease: the BISCUIT study. *PLoS One*. 2013; 8: e58825.

137. Williams BL. *et al*. Application of novel PCR-based methods for detection, quantitation, and phylogenetic characterization of *Sutterella* species in intestinal biopsy samples from children with autism and gastrointestinal disturbances. *MBio*. 2012; 3: e00261-11

138. Wang L. *et al*. Increased abundance of *Sutterella* spp. and *Ruminococcus torques* in feces of children with autism spectrum disorder. *Molecular Autism*. 2013; 4: 42.

139. Wang L. *et al*. Low relative abundances of the mucolytic bacterium *Akkermansia muciniphila* and *Bifidobacterium* spp. in feces of children with autism. *Appl Environ Microbiol*. 2011; 77: 6718–6721.

140. Png CW. *et al*. Mucolytic bacteria with increased prevalence in IBD mucosa augment in vitro utilization of mucin by other bacteria. *Am J Gastroenterol*. 2010; 105: 2420-2428.

141. Everard A. *et al*. Cross-talk between *Akkermansia muciniphila* and intestinal epithelium controls diet-induced obesity. *Proc Natl Acad Sci U S A*. 2013; 110: 9066–9071.

142. Cani PD. Crosstalk between the gut microbiota and the endocannabinoid system: impact on the gut barrier function and the adipose tissue. *Clin Microbiol Infect*. 2012; 18: 50–53.

143. Gondalia SV. *et al*. Molecular characterisation of gastrointestinal microbiota of children with autism (with and without gastrointestinal dysfunction) and their neurotypical siblings. *Autism Res*. 2012; 5: 419–427.

144. Lord RS. & Bralley JA. Clinical applications of urinary organic acids. Part 2. dysbiosis markers. *Altern Med Rev*. 2008; 13: 292–306.

145. Dodou K. & Whiteley P. In search of biomarkers – the science of metabolomics in pharmacy. *Pharmaceutical J*. 2013; 290: 512.

146. Lis AW. *et al*. Profiles of ultraviolet-absorbing components of urine from autistic children, as obtained by high-resolution ion-exchange chromatography. *Clin Chem*. 1976; 22: 1528–1532.

147. Bull G. *et al*. Indolyl-3-acryloylglycine (IAG) is a putative diagnostic urinary marker for autism spectrum disorders. *Med Sci Monit*. 2003; 9: CR422–CR425.

148. Yap IK. *et al*. Urinary metabolic phenotyping differentiates children with autism from their unaffected siblings and age-matched controls. *J Proteome Res*. 2010; 9: 2996–3004.

149. Ming X. *et al*. Metabolic perturbance in autism spectrum disorders: a metabolomics study. *J Proteome Res*. 2012; 11: 5856–5862.

150. Emond P. *et al*. GC-MS-based urine metabolic profiling of autism spectrum disorders. *Anal Bioanal Chem*. 2013; 405: 5291–5300.

151. Clayton TA. Metabolic differences underlying two distinct rat urinary phenotypes, a suggested role for gut microbial metabolism of phenylalanine and a possible connection to autism. *FEBS Lett*. 2012; 586: 956–961.

152. Zimmer C. Blog post: *When You Swallow A Grenade*. Phenomena: The Loom. National Geographic. 2012. http://phenomena.nationalgeographic.com/2012/12/18/when-you-swallow-a-grenade/

153. Goldenberg JZ. *et al.* The use of probiotics to prevent *C. difficile* diarrhea associated with antibiotic use. *Cochrane Database Syst Rev.* 2013; 5: CD006095.
154. Kronman MP. *et al.* Antibiotic exposure and IBD development among children: a population-based cohort study. *Pediatrics.* 2012; 130: e794–e803.
155. Linday LA. *Saccharomyces boulardii*: potential adjunctive treatment for children with autism and diarrhea. *J Child Neurol.* 2001; 16: 387.
156. Tung JM. *et al.* Prevention of *Clostridium difficile* infection with *Saccharomyces boulardii*: A systematic review. *Can J Gastroenterol.* 2009; 23: 817–821.
157. Posey DJ. *et al.* A pilot study of D-cycloserine in subjects with autistic disorder. *Am J Psychiatry.* 2004; 161: 2115–2117.
158. Leigh MJ. *et al.* A randomized double-blind, placebo-controlled trial of minocycline in children and adolescents with Fragile X syndrome. *J Dev Behav Pediatr.* 2013; 34: 147–155.
159. Quatermain D. *et al.* Acute but not chronic activation of the NMDA-coupled glycine receptor with D-cycloserine facilitates learning and retention. *Eur J Pharmacol.* 1994; 257: 7–12.
160. Ajamian M. *et al.* Serologic markers of Lyme Disease in children with autism. *JAMA.* 2013; 309: 1771–1773.
161. Chaudhry IB. *et al.* Minocycline benefits negative symptoms in early schizophrenia: a randomised double-blind placebo-controlled clinical trial in patients on standard treatment. *J Psychopharmacol.* 2012; 26: 1185–1193.
162. Konstantareas MM. & Homatidis S. Ear infections in autistic and normal children. *J Autism Dev Disord.* 1987; 17: 585–594.
163. Tajima-Pozo K. *et al.* Otitis and autism spectrum disorders. *BMJ Case Rep.* 2010; 2010: bcr10.2009.2351.
164. Niehus R. & Lord C. Early medical history of children with autism spectrum disorders. *J Dev Behav Pediatr.* 2006; 27(2 Suppl): S120–S127.
165. Guyonnet D. *et al.* Effect of a fermented milk containing *Bifidobacterium animalis* DN-173 010 on the health-related quality of life and symptoms in irritable bowel syndrome in adults in primary care: a multicentre, randomized, double-blind, controlled trial. *Aliment Pharmacol Ther.* 2007; 26: 475–486.
166. Critchfield JW. *et al.* The potential role of probiotics in the management of childhood autism spectrum disorders. *Gastroenterol Res Pract.* 2011; 2011: 161358.
167. Rachel WD. *et al.* Improvements in gastrointestinal symptoms among children with autism spectrum disorder receiving the Delpro® probiotic and immunomodulator formulation. *J Prob Health.* 2013; 1: 102.
168. Gough E. *et al.* Systematic review of intestinal microbiota transplantation (fecal bacteriotherapy) for recurrent *Clostridium difficile* infection. *Clin Infect Dis.* 2011; 53: 994–1002.
169. Borody TJ. *et al.* *Helicobacter pylori* eradication with doxycycline-metronidazole-bismuth subcitrate triple therapy. *Scand J Gastroenterol.* 1992; 27: 281–284.
170. Borody TJ. & Khoruts A. Fecal microbiota transplantation and emerging applications. *Nat Rev Gastroenterol Hepatol.* 2011; 9: 88–96.
171. Minot S. *et al.* The human gut virome: inter-individual variation and dynamic response to diet. *Genome Res.* 2011; 21: 1616–1625.
172. Rogers MAM. *et al.* Depression, antidepressant medications, and risk of *Clostridium difficile* infection. *BMC Medicine* 2013; 11: 121.
173. Dunn R. Blog post: *The Sieve Hypothesis: Clever Study Suggests an Alternate Explanation for the Function of the Human Stomach.* Scientific American. 2013. http://blogs.scientificamerican.com/guest-blog/2013/01/29/the-sieve-hypothesis-clever-study-suggests-an-alternate-explanation-for-the-function-of-the-human-stomach/

Chapter 6

The gluten- and casein-free (GFCF) diet and autism: episode 1

We've taken a few chapters to reach the primary reason why we assume you are reading this book. It's not that we wanted to keep you waiting or just wanted to fill space but rather that quite a few of the concepts that we've already introduced are going to crop up when talking about diet and autism. You'll note that we've split our discussions on the **gluten- and casein-free (GFCF) diet** into several episodes based on the sheer amount of material that we want to discuss and to try and keep the scientific reference list to a manageable size. Episode 1 covers the current evidence base and reported effects following dietary intervention. In episode 2 we look at some of the potential reasons how and why dietary intervention might work. In episode 3 we're going to talk about some of the practicalities of using dietary intervention in cases of autism.

It's probably accurate to say that use of GFCF dietary intervention is not uncommon with autism in mind.[174] Whether as a result of the quite numerous 'biomedical movement' comprised of those who tend to see autism as more than just the sum of its behavioural parts or as a result of another viewpoint espoused by some, suggestive that parents are just 'desperate' to do what they can for their child, dietary change is popular.

One could see how such dietary intervention might be viewed as an attractive option. Autism, to use the singular term, is a lifelong condition. There is no cure and post-diagnosis, science and medicine still offers very little universals in terms of outcome or intervention. That's a popular view.

Diet on the other hand: it's a dietary change, nothing more. So it's something within everyone's reach. It's not medicine, or more accurately it's viewed as something that doesn't involve putting 'chemicals' (remember how that word is sometimes interpreted) into the body and fits in well with an increasingly vocal consumer asking questions about their food, its safety and effects. When you boil a GFCF diet down to its source, you can still include meats, vegetables, fruits and oils into your diet: all very traditional foods we've been eating for many,

> The gluten- and casein-free (GFCF) diet remains controversial in some quarters

many years. Also, there's lots of accounts out there in cyberspace and beyond about how diet did this for a person or that for a person. And all that seemingly just because of a dietary change. We're not making light of this by the way, just pointing out some possibilities.

Without getting too philosophical, at least one of those reasons for why diet is popular – the power of the personal account - is something which has been discussed with other interventions in relation to autism too. Perhaps also a good example of how, to some people, science, and its current often generalised conclusions on a specific matter, is not necessarily an end-point but rather a part of a bigger picture. Allied to the way that many parents of children with autism have organised themselves into groups whether for support or other activities, you can perhaps see how personal accounts can be powerful and easily spread. By saying this, we're not trying to be heretics to the scientific method; just introducing it into the conversation to show how real life sometimes works.

That being said, it's inevitable that given the wide spectrum that is the autisms and the possibility that there might be more than one way for a person to arrive at the condition some people are not going to benefit from dietary implementation. The same is true of every intervention for autism. Without, hopefully, coming across as too controversial, one could perhaps also see how for those who've tried diet with their children for example, and did not see positive effects, there could likewise be a temptation to overgeneralise their alternate individual experiences of dietary intervention too. We suppose it all depends on your subjective opinions and your viewpoint. So faced with two quite vocal camps on the potential effectiveness of a GFCF diet for autism, combined with quite a lot of dogma regarding what autism is and isn't, you can perhaps see how discussions might be quite heated.

In some circles, dietary intervention is referred to, rather disparagingly one has to say, as being part of a suite of approaches known as complementary medicine. Allied to the use of the word 'unorthodox' the insinuation is that, because we aren't necessarily talking about more traditionally 'relevant' educational or behavioural or medicines therapies, diet is somehow always going to be consigned to a lower rung of the scientific ladder. We're not here to give readers some kind of scientific pros and cons overview of complementary medicine. There are plenty of other resources to go to for that. If you feel, however, that diet might actually be something which can affect physiology, behaviour and mood, though not necessarily to the same extent in everyone, then perhaps you might view dietary intervention as what it is: dietary intervention.

We've already hinted at another possible reason why the GFCF diet for autism might also have the ability to invoke considerable debate in some circles based on the links that have been made to gastrointestinal (GI) issues being present in some cases. Hopefully we've given you some food for thought on the issue of GI symptoms in relation to autism; also intersecting with factors like **leaky gut** and the gut microbiome albeit with the need for far more detailed (and controlled) research.

Allied to the point that certain GI factors have, right or wrong, been equated with certain environmental factors in relation to cases of autism, there's also the variable of who is delivering the message about dietary intervention for autism to the masses. We're not going to mention names or anything like that but will say that personalities and viewpoints can sometimes prejudice scientific debate.

There is no evidence

Throughout the history of GFCF dietary research with autism in mind, words to the effect of 'no evidence' or 'evidence lacking' have been used on quite a few occasions to try and define our knowledge and understanding of the intervention. Take for example some of the interpretations of the paper by Tim Buie,[175] a gastroenterologist who you're going to hear more about in this chapter. Quite a large quote from the abstract to his paper reviewing autism and **gluten** reads:

A variety of symptoms may be present with gluten sensitivity. Currently, there is insufficient evidence to support instituting a gluten-free diet as a treatment for autism. There may be a subgroup of patients who might benefit from a gluten-free diet, but the symptom or testing profile of these candidates remains unclear.

For some, the important parts of this passage were the words 'insufficient evidence', irrespective of the quite sensible notion that because of all that **heterogeneity** present among the autisms, there may be potential responders, just as there may be non-responders.

> Several studies have looked experimentally at the use of a GFCF diet for autism

Indeed, to say that there is insufficient evidence for a GFCF diet for cases of autism has to some extent become confused with no evidence of effect. They are not the same things and this highlights how, for whatever reason, appropriate controlled trials of the GFCF diet with autism in mind seem to have been passed over for quite a few years now as part of the autism research agenda. Therein lies the paradox: dietary intervention is a popular intervention for autism yet there is seemingly limited appetite to scientifically challenge its suggested effects. Even when groups have tried to get large-scale studies of diet and autism off the ground – look up CANDAA and autism – the response from potential funding agencies has often been less than enthusiastic.

Outside of the politics of a GFCF diet being suggested as an intervention option for autism, there is actually quite a long history of science being done on the topic down the years. As you'll see, however, the main stumbling block has been the quality of that science and its potential to introduce bias to the results reported.

The late Prof. Ann-Mari Knivsberg is perhaps the best-known name linked to investigations on the GFCF diet for autism. Ann-Mari was one of the first to explore and take seriously the anecdotal reports which were beginning to surface in the 1980s about the possibility that diet may show some link to the presentation of autism for some people. Her initial paper[176] and its follow-up[177] reflected the preliminary nature of the dietary reports being discussed. Although the research probed the potential effects of diet over a relatively long period of time looking at various facets of psychological and behavioural functions, the total number of participants included for study was small and the methodology used was an open trial. In effect, this was a study of tracking those on a diet. It was potentially biased because everyone knew whether or not they were on diet and aside from looking at those who had lapsed on to a typical diet containing gluten and **casein**, there was no control group to speak of. Nevertheless, her results indicated some potential changes in behaviour to be present among her cohort of participants coincidental to their following a GFCF diet.

The Norwegian collaboration, of which Prof. Knivsberg was a part, has similarly been involved in other, more scientifically sound studies of dietary intervention for autism. In the hierarchy of scientific evidence,[178] the results of a randomised controlled trial (RCT) represent some of the highest levels of support for a particular intervention being or not being indicated for a specific condition. Based on the assumption that random allocation to a treatment or non-treatment group should counteract selection bias, the idea is that randomly assigning a study participant to receive intervention or not should theoretically stop researchers from picking out those who they think (or know) are likely to show some positive change from the intervention in question. Within the definition of a RCT, there is also additional scope to blind either researchers or both participants and researchers as to who has been allocated to intervention or not (single- and double-blinded study), and indeed instead of just using treatment as usual as your control arm, to use various sham intervention(s) called placebo as comparators with the intervention under investigation.

> Several types of study methodology have been used to look at a GFCF diet for autism

The two RCTs on GFCF dietary intervention with involvement from Prof. Knivsberg both indicated some potential effect from the use of diet in autism. Based on following groups for one year on dietary intervention[179] and two years on dietary intervention,[180] various behavioural aspects of autism showed statistically significant changes as a function of diet. The trial, by one of the authors of this book, Whiteley and colleagues,[180] known as **ScanBrit** also included one of the largest participant groups studied to date in this area, as well as various 'gold-standard' assessment schedules covering both core and peripheral features of autism.

Both trials were single-blind studies indicating that whilst researchers were not privy to the information of who was following dietary intervention or not, participants and their families/carers did know such information. Indeed other studies of such dietary intervention have adopted a similar single-blind design[181] albeit not necessarily comparing GFCF with non-GFCF diets.

When it comes to the use of double-blind studies of the GFCF diet for autism where both researchers and participants are blinded to whether or not they receive intervention, the results are a little less straightforward with regards to a dietary effect. Elder and colleagues[182] suggested that after six weeks on diet, there were no statistically significant changes to any of the parameters that they looked at despite some anecdotal reports of changes noted by parents of study participants. It would be easy to be over-critical of the Elder study given its small participant group (N=15) and short duration of examination given the other work looking at much longer periods of study. However, one cannot discount such findings outright given that the results reported by Lucarelli and colleagues[183] looking specifically at a milk (casein) free diet in their cohort, which included a double-blind element during dietary challenge, reported an improvement after only eight weeks of dietary intervention. That this group also reported a worsening of specific behaviours when milk was reinstalled as a challenge to the diet is also of particular note.

Of related interest to the science of dietary intervention for autism is the important issue raised by Elder and colleagues on the feasibility of conducting double-blind studies in this area where both participants and researchers are blinded to diet or control group status potentially alongside a placebo arm. Unlike when testing a new medicine for a condition like autism, where the look and taste of a medicine or pill with an active ingredient can be copied to produce a dummy (placebo) pill with no medicinal effect, it's a slightly different prospect when it comes to a dietary change. Aside from different people having different preferences for the foods they enjoy eating, to trial something like a GFCF diet under double-blind conditions takes some creative thinking. We've had hints down the years of how this could be done, as in the study by Mary Goodwin and colleagues[105] which we've already talked about. So for example, both your intervention and control groups are placed on a GFCF diet. You then supplement each respective group with a set amount of gluten and casein supplement or placebo either as a food supplement or even a drink. The idea is that even though foods containing gluten and casein are removed from the diet of everyone, the supplements will, in blinded fashion, allow researchers to compare between the two groups.

Around the studies we've highlighted, there are various other scientific reports of dietary intervention for autism being examined. These have taken various forms, from further open trials such as that reported by Whiteley and colleagues[184] to individual case studies[185] to more survey-based research.[186] Interested readers are also directed to the various meta-analyses, summarising and analysing the collected data from the various studies, for further reading on this topic.[187–189]

'Insufficient evidence' is not the same as 'no evidence'

In trying to summarise the experimental evidence for any potential effect from dietary intervention for cases with autism, it is perhaps appropriate to reiterate those words 'insufficient evidence' as meaning insufficient evidence with a focus particularly on methodology, the number of participants and time on intervention. That being said, the quantity and direction of the current evidence, complete with all its failings, certainly does not imply no evidence to be present to support the notion of dietary involvement in some cases of autism.

The reported effects

One of the commonly asked questions outside of whether there is any evidence that a GFCF diet actually works is that concerning what kinds of effects it might potentially have. Whiteley and colleagues[190] summarised the main areas of behavioural 'improvement' noted across the available literature. The core dyad of symptoms (**social affect** and repetitive or stereotyped patterns of behaviour) feature throughout the evidence base. Indeed, positive changes to the use of communication such as the features of language represent one of the more consistently reported changes. Interestingly however, several peripheral features also seem to be affected by diet. This includes things like a partial amelioration of attention and concentration issues, self-injurious behaviours, motor coordination issues and hyperactive or impulsive-like behaviours.

Various behaviours have been reported to be affected by a GFCF diet

Drawing on our previous discussions on how autism is, in many cases, so much more than just the presentation of core behaviours, it is relevant that some of these 'add-on' issues also seem to be affected in some cases. We're going to talk more about whether dietary change primarily affects core or peripheral features shortly drawing on other work outside of autism.

Beyond just behavioural changes, there is some suggestion, albeit more anecdotal than scientific, that use of a GFCF diet might also affect other, more physiologically based, variables such as bowel issues and even seizure activity. Again, further discussions follow on this, bearing in mind we are not advocating a GFCF diet as a cure-all or even management tool for important and potentially life-altering conditions like **epilepsy**.

We've hinted a few times about the issue of responders and non-responders to intervention with autism in mind, and how all that heterogeneity and **comorbidity** perhaps imply that some interventions might work better for some over others. Where GFCF dietary intervention is concerned there is at the time of writing no tried and tested criteria for identifying who might be a potential dietary responder: something that Dr Buie also noted.[175] Whether as a consequence of the age groups which have generally been chosen for

It is likely that there will be 'best' and 'non responders' to a GFCF diet for cases of autism

participation in the various dietary trials or in accordance with the ethos of early intervention being 'better' in cases of autism, some commentators have suggested a relationship between chronological age and dietary effectiveness as being important. 'The younger the better' is the suggestion, although to reiterate, the scientific literature so far offers little in the way of evidence to confirm this assertion.

References

174. Le Couteur A. *et al.* Parents' and child health professionals' attitudes to dietary interventions in autism spectrum disorder (ASD): findings from a UK survey. Paper 6282. *IMFAR 2010.*
175. Buie T. The relationship of autism and gluten. *Clin Ther.* 2013; 35: 578–583.
176. Knivsberg A-M. *et al.* Dietary intervention in autistic syndromes. *Brain Dysfunct.* 1990; 3: 315–317.
177. Knivsberg A-M. *et al.* Autistic syndromes and diet: A follow-up study. *Scan J Educ Res.* 1995; 39: 223–236.
178. Brighton B. *et al.* Hierarchy of evidence: from case reports to randomized controlled trials. *Clin Orthop Relat Res.* 2003; 413: 19–24.
179. Knivsberg A-M. *et al.* A randomised, controlled study of dietary intervention in autistic syndromes. *Nutr Neurosci.* 2002; 5: 251–261.
180. Whiteley P. *et al.* The ScanBrit randomised, controlled, single-blind study of a gluten- and casein-free dietary intervention for children with autism spectrum disorders. *Nutr Neurosci.* 2010; 13: 87–100.
181. Johnson CR. *et al.* Effects of a gluten free/casein free diet in young children with autism: a pilot study. *J Dev Phys Disabil.* 2011; 23: 213–225.
182. Elder JH. *et al.* The gluten-free, casein-free diet in autism: results of a preliminary double blind clinical trial. *J Autism Dev Disord.* 2006; 36: 413–420.
183. Lucarelli S. *et al.* Food allergy and infantile autism. *Panminerva Med.* 1995; 37: 137–141.
184. Whiteley P. *et al.* A gluten-free diet as an intervention for autism and associated spectrum disorders: preliminary findings. *Autism.* 1999; 3: 45–65.
185. Hsu CL. *et al.* The effects of a gluten and casein-free diet in children with autism: a case report. *Chang Gung Med J.* 2009; 32: 459–465.
186. Pennesi CM. & Klein LC. Effectiveness of the gluten-free, casein-free diet for children diagnosed with autism spectrum disorder: based on parental report. *Nutr Neurosci.* 2012; 15: 85–91.
187. Millward C. *et al.* Gluten- and casein-free diets for autistic spectrum disorder. *Cochrane Database Syst Rev.* 2008; 2: CD003498.
188. Mulloy A. *et al.* Gluten-free and casein-free diets in the treatment of autism spectrum disorders: A systematic review. *Res Autism Spectr Disord.* 2010; 4: 328–339.
189. Mulloy A. *et al.* Addendum to 'gluten-free and casein-free diets in treatment of autism spectrum disorders: A systematic review'. *Res Autism Spectr Disord.* 2011; 5: 86–88.
190. Whiteley P. *et al.* Gluten- and casein-free dietary intervention for autism spectrum conditions. *Front Hum Neurosci.* 2012; 6: 344.

RECIPES

Apple pie with almond pastry

Now everyone can enjoy this family favourite (serves 8).

Ingredients

Pastry

170 grams of gluten-free flour mix
1 teaspoon of xanthan gum
½ teaspoon of salt
60 grams of ground almonds
110 grams of dairy-free spread
50 grams of icing sugar, sifted
2 egg yolks, beaten, and some egg white for glazing
1–2 tablespoons of cold water

Filling

3 Bramley apples
½ lemon zest and juice
60 grams of light brown sugar
½ teaspoon of cinnamon
50 grams of grated marzipan (optional)
1 teaspoon of cornflour mixed with 1 tablespoon of cold water
1 tablespoon of caster sugar

Method

Sift the flour, xanthan gum and salt into a mixing bowl. Add the ground almonds and dairy-free spread and rub in until the mixture resembles fine breadcrumbs. Stir in the sugar. Add the egg yolks to the flour mixture and mix in some water if needed. Gather together to make a soft dough. Take care not to over-mix. Wrap in cling film and chill for at least 30 minutes before rolling out with a rolling pin. After the pastry has chilled, heat the oven to 190 degrees centigrade/fan oven 170 degrees centigrade/gas mark 5. Cut off a third of the pastry and keep it wrapped while you roll out the rest, and use this to line a pie tin of approximately 20–22cm diameter and 4cm deep leaving a slight overhang over the tin. Roll the remaining third to a circle about 28cm in diameter.

Quarter, core, peel and slice the apples about 5mm thick and tip them into the bowl and toss through with the lemon juice. Gently mix in the sugar, cinnamon and lemon zest and marzipan with your hands and immediately pile high into the pastry-lined tin.

Brush a little water around the pastry rim and lay the pastry lid over the apple mixture, pressing the edges together to seal. Trim the edge carefully with a sharp knife and make 5 little slashes on top of the lid for the steam to escape. The uncooked pie can be frozen at this stage for later baking. Brush the top of the pie with the egg white and sprinkle with caster sugar. Bake for 40–45 minutes, until golden brown, then remove and let it cool for 5–10 minutes. Serve warm.

Sprinkling of nutritional science

Xanthan gum is not generally the foodstuff of choice for many people. As a thickening agent, xanthan gum is second to none, accounting for its use in various products from salad dressings to gluten-free products (providing the doughiness that such products often miss).

Rock buns/scones

A snack, a treat, tasty and sweet (makes 8–12 buns).

Ingredients

225 grams of gluten-free flour mix
75 grams of brown sugar
1 tablespoon of gluten-free baking powder
¼ teaspoon of baking soda
½ teaspoon of salt
¼ teaspoon of xanthan gum (if it's not already included in your gluten-free flour mix)
85 grams of cold dairy-free margarine
75 grams of dried fruit (raisins, cranberries)
120 grams of soya yoghurt plain or vanilla
1 egg
1–2 teaspoons of orange or lemon zest
1 teaspoon of lemon juice

Method

Preheat oven to 225 degrees centigrade/gas mark 7 and put in the tray that you are going to cook your scones on. Cut the dairy-free margarine into small pieces and place back into the fridge until needed. In a large bowl mix together the flour, brown sugar, baking powder, baking soda, salt and xanthan gum and dried fruit. Rub the spread into flour mixture until it looks like little breadcrumbs. In a separate bowl, mix together the soya yoghurt, 1 egg, 1–2 teaspoons of orange or lemon zest (optional) and lemon juice. Add the wet ingredients, leaving about 1 tablespoon or the dregs in the bottom of the bowl, to the dry ingredients to create a wet mix. Lift your heated tray out of the oven and cover with a piece of baking parchment. Spoon out your mixture on to the tray in equal-sized heaps, fairly evenly spaced between them. Brush with the left-over yoghurt and egg mixture and bake in the oven for 10–12 minutes. Cool on a wire rack. Can be served with dairy-free spread, coconut cream or jam.

Sprinkling of nutritional science

The name cranberry derives from 'crane-berry', and is a food plant of cranes and other birds. High in vitamin C as well as various flavonoids – compounds known to have anti-oxidant capability – cranberries are a refreshing addition to food. Cranberries are best known for their potential role in preventing and treating urinary tract infections (UTIs), thought to be due to their effects on bacteria such as *E. coli*.

Biscotti

Biscotti means twice baked, which makes this crunchy biscuit perfect for being dunked in your favourite hot drink (makes 16).

Ingredients

180 grams cup of gluten-free flour
30 grams of sweet rice flour
1 teaspoon of xanthan gum
½ teaspoon of baking soda
½ teaspoon of gluten-free baking powder
⅛ teaspoon of salt
110 grams of dairy-free margarine
200 grams of caster sugar
2 eggs
45 grams of flaked almonds
90 grams of dark chocolate drops (check for the dairy-free ones)
65 grams of chopped dried apricots
2 teaspoons of grated orange zest
(if you don't want to use the chocolate, pistachios and dried cranberries also work well)

Method

Mix together the gluten-free flour, sweet rice flour, xanthan gum, baking soda, baking powder and salt. Cream together dairy-free margarine and sugar and beat until fluffy, for about 5 minutes. Add in the eggs, one at a time. Stir in the nuts, fruit, chocolate chips and zest. Slowly incorporate the dry ingredients to form a soft dough. Refrigerate the dough for at least one hour or overnight. Preheat the oven to 190 degrees centigrade/gas mark 5. Lightly grease 2 oven trays and line with parchment paper. Divide the dough into 3 equal pieces. Shape each piece into a log 1½ to 2 inches thick. Place 2 logs on one sheet, and 1 log on the other sheet, leaving enough space between them for the dough to spread while baking. Bake the logs for 20 minutes. Remove from the oven and let sit for 5 to 10 minutes. Slice the logs on a slight diagonal about ¾ of an inch thick. Place the slices, cut side down, on the trays. Lower the oven temperature to 170 degrees centigrade/gas mark 3 and bake the slices for 10–12 minutes. Cool on a cooling rack. Store in an airtight container.

Sprinkling of nutritional science

Low in saturated fat but high in vitamins A and C, apricots are a flexible fruit which provide the sweet taste of summer. Also a good source of fibre, apricots are great fresh but can also be served as a dried fruit or marmalade.

Chapter 7

The gluten- and casein-free (GFCF) diet and autism: episode 2

It is the million dollar question: just how does installation of a **GFCF diet** affect behaviour and other functions in relation to cases of autism? Sadly, we're going to answer this question quickly before we go off exploring potential modes of action, by saying nobody really knows how diet might affect the presentation of autism. There's plenty of speculation and fitting together of pieces of often quite disparate pieces of evidence but that's about it. Readers are also well advised to tread carefully when coming across anyone who says that they know how dietary intervention might be working in autism.

Why might diet work?

In their (our) review article, Whiteley and colleagues[191] talked about some of the findings which may be pertinent to some dietary effect being observed in cases of autism. There are some familiar concepts already included in the review covering areas such as the **comorbidity** of **coeliac disease**[91] (discussed as a **gluten**-sensitive enteropathy) and **gut** hyperpermeability (**leaky gut**).[109] Aside from reiterating that coeliac disease is probably not significantly over-represented in autism, quite a lot of the focus has been on the so-called **gut–brain axis**.

Opioid-excess?

Like every good theory (think back to **ToM** taking on board testosterone), the issue of the gut–brain axis as being relevant to autism has been an evolving concept down the years. Initially based on the observations of psychologist/psychobiologist Jaak Panksepp,[192] who proposed a link between the brain **opioid** system and autism, the opioid-excess theory included as part of it that gut–brain axis theory which has generated quite a bit of debate.

> The opioid-excess theory proposes that gluten and casein break down into products similar to morphine

Whilst the ideas that (1) we have our own opioid system, and (2) disruption to that opioid system might manifest as autistic behaviours might seem a little far-fetched, there was some good reason to talk about this possibility. Our own brain opioid system, which includes several naturally occurring opioid-like compounds such as the **endorphins** and enkephalins, represents an important part of the human reward system; said compounds linked to feelings of wellbeing as well as analgesia (relief from pain). Buoyed by preliminary results indicating elevations in endorphin activity to be present in some cases of autism[193] the opioid-excess theory started to accumulate some interesting evidence.

Outside of the endogenous – naturally produced by the body – endorphin findings, other authors began to speculate on whether there might be exogenous – externally derived – sources of similar opioid-like compounds which might also play a role in cases of autism. The more usual opioid classes of compounds and drugs of abuse such as morphine, heroin and codeine are very, very unlikely to be taken by children with autism(!) so attention turned to a possible role for food and in particular, gluten and **casein**. Figure 7.1 illustrates the main components of the opioid-excess theory.

You're probably wondering why we are equating a powerful drug like morphine with foods which contain gluten and casein. Granted, the link might not be immediately apparent but surprisingly enough, it is known that such foods can break down into compounds which structurally, might be able to access those all-important opioid receptors similar to morphine, and begin a similar cascade of effects. Going back again to the description of proteins and **peptides**, equated as the long and short pearl necklace, it's all about peptides and the sequences generated as a consequence of digestion.

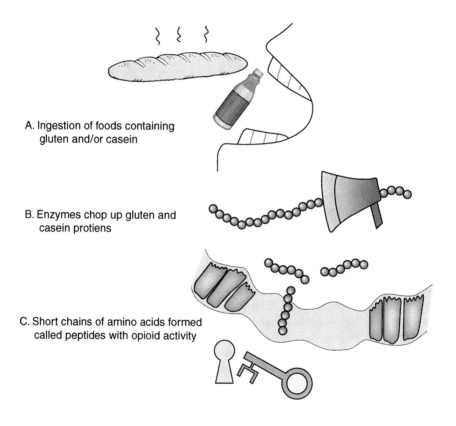

A. Ingestion of foods containing gluten and/or casein

B. Enzymes chop up gluten and casein protiens

C. Short chains of amino acids formed called peptides with opioid activity

D. Peptides traverse the gut barrirer and fit into opioid receptors

Figure 7.1 Opioid-excess theory.

Christine Zioudrou and colleagues set the ball rolling with their initial sequencing of the exorphins derived from dietary sources.[194] Followed by further confirmatory work on how both gluten and casein could be metabolised into **opioid peptides**[195,196] it's fairly well accepted these days that under the right conditions, gluten and casein can break down to opioid peptides as a consequence of digestion. Real (addictive) comfort food you might say.

Knowing then that food may be an external source of those peptides, questions then turned to whether or not they could so significantly exert an effect on behaviour and development with an end-point being a complex condition like autism. Indeed, whether such peptides are, for example, able to traverse the gut barrier and exert a central effect on the brain.

We already know that gluten peptides can gain access to the gut lining under certain conditions, as in the case of coeliac disease. Other research has hinted that opioid peptides from casein, called casomorphins, can also potentially cross the gut barrier,[197] at least under laboratory conditions. If we take into account those other findings indicating increased gut permeability in some cases of autism, one could speculate that there might be increased uptake of such peptides and other potentially active material across the gut barrier. In terms of the behavioural effects of such peptides being potentially 'causative' of autism, it's all been about extrapolating results.

The collected works of Sun and colleagues[198,199] suggested that, in rats at least, one particular **peptide** fragment from milk called beta-casomorphin 1–7 can cross the **blood-brain barrier (BBB)** which separates our brain from the rest of our body and can activate opioid receptors. Once present in the rat brain, beta-casomorphin 1–7 also correlated with some interesting behavioural changes compared to control rats. Fine if you're a rat, we hear you say, and you'd be right. Studies of real people, particularly infants, have however also suggested that problems with peptides derived from degrading cow's milk may contribute to issues with psychomotor development for example.[200] The case for a potential opioid effect is therefore not without evidence and indeed, when one takes on board the work looking at anti-opioid medicines like naltrexone for autism, the evidence base is strengthened.

Where perhaps the opioid-excess theory has come a little unstuck is with regards to how various groups have gone about seeking evidence for the presence of these exogenous peptides outside of looking in invasive biofluids. Of specific note is the controversy around the body of research looking at the possibility of detecting peptides in urine samples provided by people with autism.

Dr Karl Reichelt, another Norwegian and colleague to Ann-Mari Knivsberg, should perhaps be credited with first reporting on the possibility that biologically active peptides found in urine might be linked to cases of autism.[201] Of note were the suggestions that such peptides might also be found in other conditions such as **schizophrenia**, hinting at how the gut–brain axis, talked about with autism in mind, actually has its roots in schizophrenia and the theories of Dr F Curtis Dohan Snr. We'll be coming to his work and legacy in a later chapter.

It wasn't a completely smooth road following the initial suggestion of urinary differences in peptide patterns in cases of autism vs. asymptomatic controls. Other researchers for example, were not able to replicate the original urinary findings of the Norwegian group.[202] Indeed, the story goes that this failure to reproduce the results in cases of autism and other 'psychiatric' conditions was in part due to an issue with some of the reagents used during the original urine analyses being unwittingly replaced by certain laboratory staff. Nonetheless, subsequent papers have also highlighted the continued possibility that urinary peptides, some of dietary origin, may be present in some cases of autism.[203]

> Problems have arisen when trying to detect opioid peptides in the urine of people with autism

In more recent times, questions have turned to the methods used to undertake analysis of urine samples for the presence of urinary peptide content. We've already touched upon the science of **metabolomics** in relation to determining and measuring urine compounds thought to be of bacterial origins. The focus these days is on the quite powerful means available for elucidating compounds in urine (**MS, NMR**) compared to the less powerful methods of times gone. Where such newer technologies have been used, questions have been raised about the accuracy of some of the older findings and indeed, the entire opioid-excess hypothesis itself[204] and on more than one occasion.[205]

It is on that note that the opioid-excess theory has remained ever since.

Gut permeability and IAG?

Interestingly some of the media reporting[206] about the paper by Cass and colleagues[205] on their failure to detect urinary peptides in their cohort of children with autism reflected some of the bias against gastrointestinal issues and food potentially being related to autism. The BBC headline: 'Leaky gut autism theory doubted' seemed to bear little relation to what Cass reported on and, perhaps most revealing, cited a link between childhood vaccination and gut barrier dysfunction, which again was well outside of the remit of the Cass findings and indeed seemingly of little relevance to any potential food connection. To reiterate, Cass and colleagues looked for the presence of opioid peptides in urine. They did not measure gut permeability in their cohort.

As we've shown, subsequent research by Laura de Magistris and colleagues[109] has indicated that directly monitoring intestinal permeability 'could help to identify a subgroup of patients with autism who could benefit from a gluten-free diet'. In short, there may be a connection between leaky gut and use of dietary intervention for cases of autism. Our discussions on the research base regarding leaky gut and autism, together with the promise of more to come[111] do not require duplication. What we would like to introduce are some of the discussions on a compound detected in the urine of some people with autism and other conditions, called *trans*-indolyl-3-acryloylglycine or IAG and its potential relevance or not to gut permeability.

IAG is thought to be a derivative of the **amino acid tryptophan**. Bearing in mind our previous mention of tryptophan as being one of those aromatic amino acids which have already been talked about with autism in mind, IAG is already potentially important. Indeed, tryptophan and autism have a long research relationship stretching back some years. With autism in mind, IAG has been isolated and characterised from urine samples.[207] Detected also in elevated quantities in other conditions like Hartnup disease – a condition characterised by the poor absorption of amino acids – IAG was first described as being a potential putative marker for autism on the basis of its frequent detection in cases of autism.[208] Subsequent research did not however confirm the universal biomarker potential for IAG in relation to autism.[209]

Despite no condition-wide biomarker potential for IAG, discussions continue as to whether the presence of IAG may be reflective of other processes on-going in cases of autism. Wang and colleagues[210] (the same group who reported on the presence of *Akkermansia muciniphila*) suggested that urinary levels of IAG appeared to be elevated for those cases of autism also reporting comorbid GI disturbances.

Although still rather speculative, previous discussions on IAG, a glycine conjugate of another compound called indolylacrylic acid (IAcrA),[211] have hinted at the possibility of some action on cell membranes.[212] Speculations have turned to whether IAG may in fact be a peripheral marker for gut permeability issues[213] although still requiring greater study.

> IAG is thought to be linked to issues with gut permeability in cases of autism

Food allergy?

As in the case of coeliac disease, the word '**allergy**' is sometimes used incorrectly. In general usage, allergy has often been talked about as a catch-all description to explain a whole raft of conditions and concepts related to how we deal and interact with various facets of our environment. But that doesn't mean every condition is an allergy.

Part of the confusion about what is and isn't an allergy stems from the way allergies are categorised. The classical interpretation of an allergy is one where the body comes across something relatively benign such as food or grass pollen and mounts an IgE-mediated response to the allergen in question. IgE by the way refers to a class of **immunoglobulin** which recognises the allergen and sparks a chain of biochemical events culminating in the release of histamine (hence why we take antihistamines) along the way, including some action of mast cells which we'll talk about shortly. Probably the most serious and life-threatening condition associated with this IgE-mediated allergy (also called type 1 hypersensitivity) is anaphylaxis.

> Allergy represents the body responding to something benign

The other side of the allergy coin is the notion of a non IgE-mediated allergy. As the name suggests IgE is not implicated in these types of allergy or intolerance. Another important distinction is the time taken from exposure to an allergen to symptoms presenting. In classical allergy, symptoms generally appear rapidly after exposure. In non IgE-mediated allergy, the symptoms can manifest some time later and in the case of food, generally manifest as GI issues.[214] The question therefore arises as to whether either IgE- or non IgE-mediated food allergy could account for any effect from food, specifically foods containing gluten and casein, in cases of autism?

The short answer is all too familiar: we don't know. There is evidence that when measuring levels of immunoglobulins like IgE there doesn't appear to be any startling differences present in autism compared to asymptomatic controls.[215] That being said, there have been occasions where specific subgroups of the autism spectrum might show elevations[216] and, of course, one can't rule out more individual responses as being present (assuming testing is undertaken). Readers' attention is also drawn to research suggesting a link between the presence of an allergy-related skin condition, atopic dermatitis and overlap with the presence of autism.[217]

Building on our mention of mast cells and their role in allergy, there have been some interesting data and speculation in this area primarily from the laboratory of Prof. Theoharis Theoharides. His various studies have suggested an elevated rate of autism in cases of mastocytosis[218] – a rare condition characterised by elevated levels of mast cells gathering in the body. Mast cells, by the way, are cells which when activated during allergy spill out their contents which includes histamine, **serotonin** and chemicals called **cytokines**, which you'll hear more about later. As a consequence of the less than apparent evidence of any involvement from

> Traditional IgE-mediated allergy is unlikely to account for any dietary effect in autism

IgE-mediated allergy, speculations have turned to whether other factors might influence mast cell activation in cases of autism.[219]

Whether other less classical allergy mechanisms might pertain to issues with food in cases of autism has been the topic of some discussion. Our previous description of the trial of a milk-free diet conducted by Lucarelli and colleagues[183] did not include their reports on elevated levels of other immunoglobulins, IgA, IgG and IgM, specifically in relation to casein. Also of great interest are the reports that the immune response to foods such as dairy products in cases of autism might be able to interact with responses to other antigens such as bacterial infections and promote **autoimmunity**.[220] We should also mention the report of **food protein–induced enterocolitis syndrome (FPIES)**– a severe GI food hypersensitivity – appearing in cases of autism.[221]

What is clear from the evidence available thus far is that classical food allergy, IgE-mediated food allergy, is probably not going to be able to account for any direct effect of dietary change in cases of autism. There is more promising research emerging from the non IgE-mediated allergy domain specifically with IgG antibodies to gliadin in mind for example but, even there, one has to be slightly cautious in linking physiological and biochemical findings back to the complexities of presented behaviours.

Carbohydrates?

Have we got it all wrong? Some people might say that this book is wrong. But our question is specifically focused on our highlighting gluten and casein as being the suspected culprits behind the changes (tentatively) reported in the science literature on diet and autism so far. Is there a bigger issue present in cases of autism outside of just proteins and **peptides** in relation to things like **carbohydrates**?

Apparently the most plentiful class of compound found in living organisms, carbohydrates (carbs) or saccharides, represent a great energy source for the human body primarily as a function of their glucose-providing properties. You've probably heard the terms 'simple' and 'complex' carbohydrates being used to denote how quickly the energy is digested and released from these different types of carbs and how we should all be aiming to eat more complex carbohydrate rich foods like certain fruits, vegetables and whole grains. The theory is that unlike very simple carbs called monosaccharides, the more complex carbs (di-, oligo- and poly-saccharides) release their energy over a longer, more sustained period, which has important effects on glucose (blood sugar) levels and available energy.

> Carbohydrates are a rich energy source for the body

Foods which contain gluten or casein can also be categorised as carbohydrates. Milk and dairy products contain galactose and **lactose**, mono and disaccharides respectively (although generally more lactose is present). Cereal produce included as whole grains which contain gluten are also tagged as complex carbohydrates, although it should be remembered that gluten itself is a protein not a carbohydrate.

If one thinks of the body as a machine, it makes good sense to evolve the mechanisms to digest carbohydrates and unlock their energy rich sugars as an alternative fuel source to protein and fats. The excessive availability of this rich fuel source in our modern-day world has however also been associated with various conditions and diseases, not least the increasing prevalence of **diabetes**.

The body uses various enzymes to break down carbohydrates to unlock their energy-rich sugars. Similar in principle to the chopping up of proteins into **peptides** and eventually **amino acids**, the enzyme amylase is an important starting part of that digestive process which begins even before we swallow our food. Thereafter a variety of carbohydrase – the collective name for enzymes degrading carbohydrates – go to work in our gut, depending on the carbohydrate fragment they are trying to digest. Examples include lactase which breaks down lactose and sucrase, involved in the conversion of sucrose to fructose.

Down the years there have been various suggestions that levels of some of these enzymes, or the genes which control production of these enzymes, might not be optimal in cases of autism. Whether due to a more generalised issue with digestion and the conditions in the GI tract not being conducive to efficient digestion (the acidity of the gut, the need for specific chemicals to aid digestion, etc.), there is a small but important bank of evidence suggestive of issues with carbohydrate metabolism in cases of autism.

We've already mentioned Dr Tim Buie in our discussions on the science behind a GFCF diet. Buie and colleagues have to some degree led the scientific discussions about issues with carbohydrate metabolism in autism. To quote from one of their papers[222]: 'Lactase deficiency not associated with intestinal **inflammation** or injury is common in autistic children'. This observation was based on their evaluations of nearly 200 children with autism, and in particular, their findings in relation to the metabolism of lactose, the sugar from milk and dairy products.

Actually to give fair dues where required, the paper by Rafail Kushak which included Buie on the authorship list was to some degree standing on the shoulders of giants in the shape of the even earlier report by Dr Karoly Horvath and colleagues.[223] Horvath similarly reported 'low intestinal carbohydrate digestive enzyme activity' in their smaller participant group but at a surprisingly similar rate to that detailed by Kushak.

Another potentially important piece to the whole **carbohydrate** metabolism in autism puzzle was discussed in a paper by Brent Williams and colleagues.[224] The same authorship group who described those interesting *Sutterella* bacteria findings, Williams *et al.* conducted a two-purpose study looking at the gut microbiota in cases of autism alongside gene expressions in various parts of the gut coding for carbohydrate enzymes. What they found was potentially very revealing in that messenger **RNA (mRNA)** – the genetic source material for building proteins and enzymes – for disaccharidase (carbohydrate) enzymes was markedly decreased in their autism group in one part of the gut examined. This covered several types of carbohydrase including sucrase isomaltase, maltase glucoamylase, and lactase and implied that there may be issues in the manufacture of these enzymes. In quite a few cases of their relatively small participant group mRNA levels were reduced governing all three enzymes. They also reported issues with the transport of carbohydrates through the gut barrier. Similar findings on a master 'transcriptional regulator' called CDX_2 suggested by Williams to be a predictor of mRNA expression of the carbohydrate enzymes have also been reported by Stephen Walker and colleagues[118] during their examination of inflammatory bowel features in cases of autism.

> Issues with the digestion of carbohydrates have been detected in cases of autism

Going back to the collected work looking at the gut microbiome in cases of autism, Williams and colleagues also hinted that issues with carbohydrate metabolism may alter what 'food' is available for the multitude of hungry bacterial mouths to feed on. This then allows certain types of bacteria to flourish and others not so where usually, adequate **carbohydrate** digestion would maintain a balance in the bacterial species to be present.

Whilst we have touched very generally on the examination of bacterial metabolites in urine in cases of autism, there is a wider literature that suggests that alterations are present as a function of differing bacteria producing different chemicals appearing in different biofluids. Lynn Wang and colleagues[225] yet again show up on the research radar and their findings of elevations in certain short chain fatty acids and ammonia in stool samples from children with autism. They concluded that increases in such products may imply differences with the fermentation – similar to the process of making beer and wine – in the gut as a consequence of the bacteria present and predominating. Indeed one specific short chain fatty acid called **propionic acid** is currently receiving quite a lot of research attention in relation to autism from certain groups.[226]

We know there's quite a lot to take in from this section. To boil it down, the suggestion is that there is some genetic vulnerability to inadequate carbohydrate digestion which may subsequently impact on the balance of types of bacteria present in the gut and, onwards, on their effect on the host. Throw in issues with gut permeability and what that might mean in terms of bacterial translocation or other compounds leeching outside of the comforts of the gut, and there are several issues which require further investigation.

In terms of the influence of **antibiotics** and probiotics on what bacteria may or may not be present in the gut, the implication is that such measures will only have short-term effects as long as issues with carbohydrate metabolism continue the cycle. As we have already discussed, removing foods which contain gluten and casein from the diet would potentially reduce total **carbohydrate** load and hence not 'overwork' what **enzyme** activity might still function. Others have suggested going further as shown by the various discussions on the **specific carbohydrate diet (SCD)**[227] – removing all starches and complex carbohydrates – and a further extension, the **gut and psychology syndrome (GAPS) diet**,[228] focused also on modifying the gut microbiota by way of probiotics and use of fermented foods. Without wishing to provide any endorsement, one can perhaps see the logic on the basis of the small but important evidence base presented so far.

> Problems with carbohydrate digestion could account for the effects of a GFCF diet in autism

Enzymes?

Quite a common theme across several of the explanations put forward to account for the effects reported following use of a GFCF diet in cases of autism have stressed a role for enzymes. Enzymes, in this role, disassemble **proteins/peptides** or carbohydrates into simpler elements onwards to allowing us to derive nutrition from them. As we've discussed, enzymes are controlled by our genes, but they're also to some degree affected by their working conditions. For enzymes working in the gut, there are some important variables which can affect their release and functioning, not least the acidity of the GI tract. In particular, those enzymes which are hardened to work in the very acidic region that is the **stomach** are quite sensitive chemicals.

> Issues with enzymes used to digest food have been reported in cases of autism

There is a small body of research literature which has inquired whether outside of limiting the foods which normally require digestion by certain enzymes it may also be possible to artificially supplement the enzymes themselves.[229] Again with no endorsement intended, Brudnak and colleagues[230] hinted during an observational trial that there may be some merit in further examination of supplemental digestive enzymes. Complemented by other on-going research on preparations such as CM-AT[231] a possible role for enzyme and enzyme replacement intervention for autism remains a possibility. That being said, there is still debate in this area regarding which enzymes might potentially be at fault and whether such an intervention alone is enough to affect presented symptoms. Indeed, not all results produced so far have been entirely positive.[232]

Reflections

By no means are we suggesting that our discussions on how diet might work in cases of autism should be taken as an exhaustive list. They merely represent the areas where science has done a little bit of investigation and offered some evidence for or against a particular idea or hypothesis. Neither should readers assume that only one mechanism might pertain per case of autism. As we've said before, a diagnosis of autism is seemingly protective of nothing when it comes to comorbidity and that includes the presence of multiple comorbidities.

> Different reasons for the effects of a GFCF diet in autism might pertain to different people

As interest in dietary intervention, right or wrong, grows we envisage that further advances will be made to delineate subgroups of potential responders and non-responders to dietary intervention and, hopefully, uncover further information to account for the reports on diet and autism. With all of these options vying to account for why diet might work, the important issue remains that for any theory to shine it must be able to comprehensively account not just for physiology but also for the complexity that is behaviour and even cognition: in essence, to truly demonstrate a gut–brain or a bacteria–brain or an immune–brain link as being pertinent to autism.

In a later chapter, we are going to highlight various investigations being done in other areas of behaviour and psychiatry with a dietary theme running through, nearly all of which have some potential link to cases of autism. With that in mind, we're going to end this chapter with a question: does dietary intervention act on the core symptoms of autism or merely represents an effect on comorbidity peripherally affecting core symptoms?

References

191. Whiteley P. *et al.* How could a gluten- and casein-free diet ameliorate symptoms associated with an autism spectrum condition? *Autism Insights.* 2010; 2: 39–53.
192. Panksepp J. A neurochemical theory of autism. *Trends in Neurosciences.* 1979; 2: 174–177.
193. Gillberg C. *et al.* Endorphin activity in childhood psychosis. Spinal fluid levels in 24 cases. *Arch Gen Psychiatry.* 1985; 42: 780–783.
194. Zioudrou C. *et al.* Opioid peptides derived from food proteins. The exorphins. *J Biol Chem.* 1979; 254: 2446–2449.
195. Brantl V. *et al.* Novel opioid peptides derived from casein (beta-casomorphins). I. Isolation from bovine casein peptone. *Hoppe Seylers Z Physiol Chem.* 1979; 360: 1211–1216.
196. Fukudome S. & Yoshikawa M. Opioid peptides derived from wheat gluten: their isolation and characterization. *FEBS Lett.* 1992; 296: 107–111.

197. Sienkiewicz-Szłapka E. *et al.* Transport of bovine milk-derived opioid peptides across a Caco-2 monolayer. *Int Dairy J* 2009; 19: 252–257.

198. Sun Z. *et al.* β-casomorphin induces Fos-like immunoreactivity in discrete brain regions relevant to schizophrenia and autism. *Autism.* 1999; 3: 67–83.

199. Sun Z. & Cade JR. A peptide found in schizophrenia and autism causes behavioral changes in rats. *Autism.* 1999; 3: 85–95.

200. Kost NV. *et al.* Beta-casomorphins-7 in infants on different type of feeding and different levels of psychomotor development. *Peptides.* 2009; 30: 1854–1860.

201. Reichelt KL. *et al.* Biologically active peptide-containing fractions in schizophrenia and childhood autism. *Adv Biochem Psychopharmacol.* 1981; 28: 627–643.

202. Le Couteur A. *et al.* Infantile autism and urinary excretion of peptides and protein-associated peptide complexes. *J Autism Dev Disord.* 1988; 18: 181–190.

203. Pedersen OS. *et al.* Serotonin uptake stimulating peptide found in plasma of normal individuals and in some autistic urines. *J Pept Res.* 1999; 53: 641–646.

204. Hunter LC. *et al.* Opioid peptides and dipeptidyl peptidase in autism. *Dev Med Child Neurol.* 2003; 45: 121–128.

205. Cass H. *et al.* Absence of urinary opioid peptides in children with autism. *Arch Dis Child.* 2008; 9: 745–750.

206. BBC News: *Leaky gut autism theory doubted.* 17 March 2008. http://news.bbc.co.uk/1/hi/health/7300327.stm (accessed July 2013).

207. Anderson RJ. *et al.* Identification of indolyl-3-acryloylglycine in the urine of people with autism. *J Pharm Pharmacol.* 2002; 54: 295–298.

208. Bull G. *et al.* Indolyl-3-acryloylglycine (IAG) is a putative diagnostic urinary marker for autism spectrum disorders. *Med Sci Monit.* 2003; 9: CR422–425.

209. Wright B. *et al.* Is the presence of urinary indolyl-3-acryloylglycine associated with autism spectrum disorder? *Dev Med Child Neurol.* 2005; 47: 190–192.

210. Wang L. *et al.* Is urinary indolyl-3-acryloylglycine a biomarker for autism with gastrointestinal symptoms? *Biomarkers.* 2009; 14: 596–603.

211. Marklová E. Where does indolylacrylic acid come from? *Amino Acids.* 1999; 17: 401–413.

212. Bell JG. *et al.* Red blood cell fatty acid compositions in a patient with autistic spectrum disorder: a characteristic abnormality in neurodevelopmental disorders? *Prostaglandins Leukot Essent Fatty Acids.* 2000; 63: 21–25.

213. Shattock P. & Whiteley P. Biochemical aspects in autism spectrum disorders: updating the opioid-excess theory and presenting new opportunities for biomedical intervention. *Expert Opin Ther Targets.* 2002; 6: 175–183.

214. Jyonouchi H. Non-IgE mediated food allergy. *Inflamm Allergy Drug Targets.* 2008; 7: 173–180.

215. Heuer L. *et al.* Reduced levels of immunoglobulin in children with autism correlates with behavioral symptoms. *Autism Res.* 2008; 1: 275–283.

216. Magalhães ES. *et al.* Immune allergic response in Asperger syndrome. *J Neuroimmunol.* 2009; 216: 108–112.

217. Yaghmaie P. *et al.* Mental health comorbidity in patients with atopic dermatitis. *J Allergy Clin Immunol.* 2013; 131: 428–433.

218. Theoharides TC. Autism spectrum disorders and mastocytosis. *Int J Immunopathol Pharmacol.* 2009; 22: 859–865.

219. Theoharides TC. Is a subtype of autism an allergy of the brain? *Clin Ther.* 2013; 35: 584–591.

220. Vojdani A. *et al.* Antibodies to neuron-specific antigens in children with autism: possible cross-reaction with encephalitogenic proteins from milk, *Chlamydia pneumoniae* and Streptococcus group A. *J Neuroimmunol.* 2002; 129: 168–177.

221. Jyonouchi H. *et al.* Immunological characterization and transcription profiling of peripheral

blood (PB) monocytes in children with autism spectrum disorders (ASD) and specific polysac-charide antibody deficiency (SPAD): case study. *J Neuroinflammation.* 2012; 9: 4.

222. Kushak RI. *et al.* Intestinal disaccharidase activity in patients with autism: effect of age, gender, and intestinal inflammation. *Autism.* 2011; 15: 285–294.

223. Horvath K. *et al.* Gastrointestinal abnormalities in children with autistic disorder. *J Pediatr.* 1999; 135: 559–563.

224. Williams BL. *et al.* Impaired carbohydrate digestion and transport and mucosal dysbiosis in the intestines of children with autism and gastrointestinal disturbances. *PLoS One.* 2011; 6: e24585.

225. Wang L. *et al.* Elevated fecal short chain fatty acid and ammonia concentrations in children with autism spectrum disorder. *Dig Dis Sci.* 2012; 57: 2096–2102.

226. Frye RE. *et al.* Unique acyl-carnitine profiles are potential biomarkers for acquired mito-chondrial disease in autism spectrum disorder. *Transl Psychiatry.* 2013; 3: e220.

227. Gottschall E. *Breaking the vicious cycle: Intestinal health through diet.* 1994; Kirkton Press.

228. Campbell-McBride N. *Gut and Psychology Syndrome.* 2004; Medinform.

229. Webb S. Drugmakers dance with autism. *Nature Biotechnology.* 2010; 28: 772–774.

230. Brudnak MA. *et al.* Enzyme-based therapy for autism spectrum disorders – is it worth another look? *Med Hypotheses.* 2002; 58: 422–428.

231. Fallon J. & Heil M. The role of a biomarker in the double blind placebo-controlled study of CM-AT in children with autistic disorder ages 3–8. Paper 11994. *IMFAR 2012.*

232. Munasinghe SA. *et al.* Digestive enzyme supplementation for autism spectrum disorders: a double-blind randomized controlled trial. *J Autism Dev Disord.* 2010; 40: 1131–1138.

RECIPES

Strawberry ice cream

Making dairy-free ice cream can be tricky because it is the fat content of the dairy which makes it scoopable. The liquor, gelatine and coconut fat are added to give flavour but also help it to texture as expected (makes approx. 560mls/1 pint).

Ingredients

500 grams of fresh strawberries
1 tablespoon of caster sugar
1 teaspoon of salt
450 millilitres of strawberry liquor
2 egg yolks
60 grams of sugar
1 tin of full fat coconut milk, chilled
50 grams of creamed coconut
1 sheet of gelatine

Method

Preheat the oven to 190 degrees centigrade, gas mark 5. Line a baking tray with parchment. Slice the strawberries and lay them out on the tray. Sprinkle with the sugar and salt and roast in the middle of the oven for about 25 minutes. Remove from the oven and allow to cool completely (this stage can be done in advance and then stored in the fridge for up to two days). Once chilled add the strawberry liquor. To make the ice cream custard base place some water in a fairly small pan with a glass bowl over the top so it doesn't touch the water. Add the egg yolks and sugar to the bowl and beat over the water till the sugar melts and it becomes smooth and shiny. This should take about 5 minutes. Add the coconut milk and creamed coconut and whisk to combine and allow to warm. It should thicken slightly so that it will coat the back of the spoon. Remove from the heat and allow to cool completely. Place the sheet of gelatine in some cold water until it becomes soft. Remove and squeeze out the excess water and place in a dry pan and allow it to melt, this should only take 30 seconds. Mix the gelatine into the custard, add the strawberry mixture and place in an ice cream maker and churn according to the instructions. Transfer to a freezable container and freeze until firm.

Sprinkling of nutritional science

Strawberries are the poster fruit of the summer season because of their appearance, taste and aroma. Bursting with vitamin C as well as an array of health-providing chemicals and nutrients, a serving of strawberries will revitalise many sweets and puddings. According to some research, strawberries may also be an elixir of life in view of their positive effects on wrinkles.

Raspberry brûlée

Light refreshing fruity dessert . . . perfect for summer days (serves 4).

Ingredients

320 grams of raspberries
250 grams soya or other dairy-free plain yoghurt
3 tablespoons of honey
1 teaspoon of vanilla extract
2 teaspoons of Demerara sugar
4 brûlée dishes or small ramekins

Method

Divide evenly the raspberries between the dishes. Mix the honey and vanilla into the yoghurt and divide between the dishes, gently mixing into raspberries. Lightly sprinkle with sugar and then either use a blow torch or hot grill to melt the sugar.

Sprinkling of nutritional science

Think vanilla and most people will think vanilla ice cream. There is, however, so much more to this flavouring derived from an orchid, as shown in its various uses in the food, perfumery and pharmaceutical industries. As an oil, vanilla has been suggested to possess a sedative quality but the active ingredient, vanillin, is where it's all thought to happen as science looks to its anti-inflammatory properties in conditions such as inflammatory bowel diseases. This on top of suggestions that vanillin might just help us to deal with pain too.

Frozen banana pudding

A great alternative texture to serve banana.

Ingredients per person

1 frozen banana
3 tablespoons of soya yoghurt
¼ teaspoon of cinnamon
1 pinch of 100 per cent stevia or 1 tablespoon of agave nectar or honey

Method

Peel the banana, chop and place in a freezer bag and freeze for at least 2 hours. Place all the ingredients in a blender making sure the blades are covered (if not you might need more yoghurt blended thoroughly). Serve immediately. You can add toppings of your choice, such as fruit, nuts or dairy-free chocolate chips.

Sprinkling of nutritional science

Most people will be unfamiliar with agave nectar and its sweet-tasting properties. Derived from the agave plant, agave nectar is sweeter than sugar yet possesses a lower glycaemic load than normal sugar.

Part III

The practical part, and more

Chapter 8

The gluten- and casein-free (GFCF) diet and autism: episode 3

In line with the saying 'nothing about us without us' we should have perhaps said this sooner, but this book is intended as a 'practical guide for families and professionals' and as authors we also very much welcome those diagnosed with an autism spectrum condition to read our summaries of the collected experimental work on **GFCF diets** and autism. Our use of the word 'practical' is to some extent already covered by the inclusion of all those tasty recipes that you've seen dotted around this book. In this chapter we're also going a little further, with the emphasis on 'practical' and some discussions on food and the ways and means you might be able to make mealtimes less hassled and more fun.

In this chapter we're also going to further explore the various sensory issues which have been described in cases of autism. We're going to talk about how food intake and eating patterns could potentially be affected by such sensory issues and how these can quite significantly impact on how well interventions like the GFCF diet are for example, received. Again, we don't claim to have some intimate insight into all these processes. Like everything seemingly related to autism, there are quite a lot of individual differences to be present as shown by the example of the N = 1. People are different and what might work for one family or person might not work for others.

We're also going to talk about how one might go about trialling a GFCF diet and some of the potential pitfalls to be on the look out for. We should perhaps also say that we're not completely giving up on physiology and biochemistry insofar as our discussing nutrition and autism with a focus on **vitamins** and **minerals** in light of how implementation of a restrictive diet might potentially affect such intakes.

It might be a good time for us also to reiterate our caveat about **not giving medical advice in this book** and stress how many useful people there are out there to help and provide advice to people with autism and their parents/carers about autism, mealtimes and the various relationships with food. That and understanding that the tips we provide in this chapter are not meant to be implemented all at once but rather spread out over time.

Early infant feeding

We've already mentioned how the description of autism provided by Dr Leo Kanner in his 1943 paper[31] detailed so much more than just overt behaviour. By our reckoning, 6 of the original 11 children talked about by Kanner were also described as presenting with feeding issues, many of which seemed to start quite early in infancy. The descriptions ranged from the presence of 'early vomiting' to 'severe feeding difficulty from the beginning of life' to 'having to be tube-fed'. Of course, this was just a case description, and such feeding issues are by no means exclusive to children later diagnosed with autism. That being said, one might reasonably ask, knowing what kind of things infants are normally fed during their earliest years and the combined literature suggestive of a possible link between diet and autism, whether these findings might represent something worthy of more investigation. Indeed one question we might have had for Kanner's original cohort would be to ask how many might have presented with **lactose** intolerance in view of figures[222] previously discussed?

Although currently a little sparse, there are indications from the research literature that some groups are taking seriously the early extra-behavioural presentation of early autism. Barnevik Olsson and

> Potentially important food-related clues are present in the early descriptions of autism

colleagues,[233] for example, reported on how early feeding issues as part of a wider group of regulatory issues, such as sleep, did seem to be more frequently reported for children in early childhood who were later diagnosed with autism. Other groups including one of the authors of this book have detailed similar findings,[234] even suggesting that there may be differences in diagnostic groupings according to the presence of such early feeding issues. In short, Kanner's observations might not necessarily just have been a chance association. One must, however, view these findings as part of a more general picture in terms of the manifestations of early feeding issues in other areas of child development. Learning and physical disabilities are often associated with feeding issues.

Food glorious food?

The topic of food and autism, outside of any special dietary connection, has received its fair share of coverage down the years. Whether discussing the various likes and dislikes of children with autism, the complicating issues of rituals and routines, or with sensory issues in mind, food and eating can be an intricate business when it comes to autism.

Going back to some of our very early discussions in this book on how autism is not a failure to develop and the very **heterogeneous** nature of child development, it is important to understand that children, particularly very young children, generally are not perfect eaters irrespective of a diagnosis of autism or not. OK, some children are; some kids will eat almost anything put in front of them from their earliest days without even batting an eyelid. But they tend to be the minority. Most parents will more commonly identify with some degree of pickiness when it comes to food choices (particularly for fruits and vegetables) and recount stages of 'faddy' eating. Indeed such food issues when they occur can be a source of significant familial stress.

It is, however, the degree and intensity with which such feeding issues can manifest in cases of autism that perhaps set them apart from other reports of feeding issues as almost being a developmental stage in child development. Quite a few parents of children with autism that we've been in contact with describe how their child's eating lives are governed by issues such as food refusal and type and texture sensitivity. It might be the smallest thing which sends a mealtime into a spin. One food touching another, the food being served on a different plate from the usual one, even whether one specific food component has been under- or over-cooked a small degree, have all been mentioned.

It's the taste

Several years ago one of our author group published a commentary on feeding patterns and autism.[235] It wasn't based on a spectacularly great investigation in terms of the methodology used, it has to be said; it was, rather, a study which randomly picked out 100 children diagnosed with an autism spectrum condition and asked their parents about their children's eating habits and feeding patterns.

The qualitative data which was received suggested a few interesting trends to be present in this group. Over 8 out of 10 parents reported that their child's core diet was fairly restrictive. Some described the desire of their children to maintain this restrictive diet as bordering on an 'obsession'. Quite a few parents also detailed how stressful the situation could become if this restrictive diet was somehow modified: in extreme cases resulting in what might be called 'challenging behaviours' such as tantrums or aggression. In other instances, food was described as actually having the ability to invoke a physiological reaction such as retching or vomiting when seeing or smelling a newly presented menu item.

Quite a few parents also noted that their children's food choices seemed to be based on their accompanying sensory issues. Some children seemed to prefer only very dry and often quite bland foods, often with a crispy or crunchy texture. For others it was the opposite: in some cases it was almost life on a puréed diet. Other children were extremely adverse to lumpy foods. Some children really, really enjoyed the taste and sensation of hot, spicy, flavoursome foods like curry or similar dishes. In other cases, children were drinking undiluted cordial drinks. Packaging was also an issue brought up by some parents. The food preferences of some children seemed to be driven more by the colour and presentation of the food packaging than its actual taste or appearance.

> Various food-related issues have been reported in cases of autism

Tips of the trade

Our previous list of food-related issues reported present in cases of autism is not by any means meant to be exhaustive. Neither are we suggesting that everyone with autism will have a food issue or the same patterns of food issues, despite the quite high percentage reporting in our previous cohort. In accordance with the ethos of this book, importantly including the important concept of **comorbidity**, the first question that anyone should ask when food issues are present is whether or not this is part of the presentation of autism or reflective of something else.

There are quite a few potential factors which could figure under that 'something else' heading. We've already talked about one or rather several possibilities with our discussions on GI issues in relation to autism. In amongst the various **gut** issues that can influence feeding behaviours, conditions like **gastro–oesophageal reflux disease (GORD)** – characterised by **stomach** acid ascending into the **oesophagus**, or reflux – can be associated with food refusal for example. Similarly, other conditions with a reflux element to them may also be associated with feeding issues. Jarocka-Cyrta and colleagues[236] described a case of eosinophilic oesophagitis comorbid to the presentation of autism as being a likely source of feeding difficulties. Formal guidance on how comorbid GI issues might manifest as feeding problems in cases of autism is available.[237]

Physical comorbidity affecting how food is digested is perhaps only one part of the issue, however. We've talked about how GI comorbidity cannot necessarily be separated from other conditions such as the presence of anxiety and sensory issues, a point which has been reiterated by other authors.[238] One could perhaps see how a learned response to pain associated with eating, for example, could turn an isolated situation into something very much more chronic and long-term. A similar situation could be envisaged in other areas where for example a chronic functional bowel habit problem like constipation could seriously affect the experience of going to the toilet. Prompt resolution of any accompanying GI issues which may impact on feeding behaviour is therefore of great importance.

> Rule out physical comorbidity first as accounting for any food or eating issues in autism

Whilst we're talking about comorbidity and autism, we should also perhaps mention about how other psychiatric comorbidity can also impact on feeding and the relationship with food. Depression is something we've talked about as being potentially present in some cases of autism. Stewart and colleagues[239] described how depression might manifest in cases of autism including its presentation related to feeding issues. One can see how various other comorbidity might also produce similar problems with food.

Motor issues are also something to consider when talking about autism and feeding patterns and habits. All those potential fine and gross motor issues may very well have the ability to affect things like the use of cutlery and other utensils. So something as seemingly trivial as coordinating hand movements to pick up food with a fork or cut food with a knife could be affected and have an impact. Similarly, the use of various muscle groups to chew and swallow food might also be looked at from the point of view of motor issues and potentially impacting on feeding behaviours.[240] We'll reiterate the value of a good **OT** where such issues potentially pertain.

And then we have the effects of some of the medicines used to manage either core or add-on conditions which can present alongside autism. We don't really want to go through a long list of medications which are known to affect appetite and feeding behaviours specifically with autism in mind, but certainly side-effects of such medicines should always be kept in mind.

Learning and the associated issue of unlearning behaviours represents an important part of any strategy to manage feeding problems if and when they arise. The emphasis is on maintaining a consistent approach; sticking to your guns, whilst all the while being mindful of how change has to be a partnership process. Don't expect everything to change overnight. Learning is a gradual process and small steps are often easier to put in place and it also helps the person at the centre of the process to see such a gradual transformative process in action.

So then, some more questions to ask yourself when confronted with someone with autism who has feeding issues starting with: is the child / person actually hungry? It may sound a little bit obvious but the truth of the matter is that not everyone experiences hunger at the same time or perhaps in the same way. Yes, we've installed these very convenient times of the day when we eat breakfast, lunch and dinner but people aren't clocks and not everyone might be in tune to such societal demands. Take breakfast for example. There's an assumption that we break our sleeping fast (breakfast) with this meal. But then that implies that someone has had a good night's sleep and wakes with the feeding urge. Suppose that someone does not live within these boundaries. That for whatever reason, a person's body clock – the circadian rhythm – does not seem to adhere to the 24-hour cycle but is instead a little out of sync with the rest of the world. There is some evidence to suggest that such a position can and does manifest in some people with autism. The self-correction of the circadian cycle which is usually undertaken does not seem to happen: the result being that some children/adults with autism seem only in phase with day and night for a part of their lives. Just imagine how this might also affect the feeding regime. For this reason, and assuming that a change can be practically made, think about altering mealtimes, for example at the weekend, to see how this might affect eating patterns and behaviour.

> Hunger is linked to the function of our body clock

Allied to the question of whether someone is actually hungry or not is the issue of snacking. We define snacking as basically any food which is consumed outside of the set meal times. Everyone snacks. Everyone at sometime gets and gives into those hunger pangs. The question to think about is how often snacking occurs and to what extent snacking turns into a meal of itself. Under certain conditions, snacking is actually an integral part of autism or rather some approaches to managing autism.

The use of food as a reinforcer of behaviour in models such as **applied behavioural analysis (ABA)** is testament to that fact. It might only be a small food 'treat' on each reinforcing occasion but depending on the frequency of its use, one can see how a child might become a serial snacker. The chances are also that it's probably not going to be a vegetable or fruit reinforcement either. The obvious thing to say would be to minimise snacking wherever possible or at least try and avoid giving snacks 1 or 2 hours before a meal. If you really have to use it, use small portions of snack food and limit the types of food to something like pieces of fruit.

> Try and limit any snacking in between meal times

The question of where a person eats their food is also something to consider which might affect their eating habits and patterns. Realising that people don't usually eat their set meals at the same venue, one might ask the question of whether the surrounding environment can affect mealtime behaviour. Most parents will already know what happens when something like a favourite TV programme is left on and watched by a child during their meal. The shift in attention from what's on the plate in front of them to the goings-on of that favourite cartoon character can noticeably affect eating behaviour. The same can very much pertain where autism is present.

Having already alluded to the sensory issues which can and do present alongside cases of autism, one might also reasonably assume that more subtle environmental factors might also affect eating behaviour. This could be an issue of the ambient temperature of the room or the presence of artificial lights, the sound and flickering from which have on quite a few occasions been suggested to affect some people on the autism spectrum. If eating with others, children or adults, one might also question whether this has a positive or negative effect particularly where children may be eating with younger siblings who are rarely quiet at the dinner table and where siblings are in proximity to the child. Try altering where you eat. It might sound like a chore to start with but move the dinner table around the house and see what happens. Experiment.

> The eating environment might be an important variable

The pace of modern life often means that we don't perhaps pay as much attention to the presentation of our food as we should. When we speak about presentation, we're not just talking about the food on our plates, but also the 'table environment'. Indeed, how this might also potentially affect the relationship a person has with food. Again it might sound trivial but looking at what is present on the dinner table might be something to consider when faced with a child or adult with autism presenting with feeding issues. So the tablecloth – its pattern or design – could be a source of distraction. The chair a person sits on, the placemat on which their food is served, the plate and the cutlery. Where parents are seated in relation to their children (normally this should be opposite or next to the child), and even a small detail like whether water is served with the meal or not, could conceivably affect whether a meal is consumed or not.

We've already mentioned how some people with autism seem to show specific preferences for 'types' of food, thought to be related to those sensory issues which we continue to talk about. Food presentation is quite a big variable for any child when making their decisions to eat or not. Any ritual or routine which stresses that, for example, this food should be next to this food, or that food should not be touching that food, can be the difference between a meal being eaten or not. Parents will probably already know what their child does and doesn't like in terms of how food is presented and, we assume, will have already communicated to other places such as school or residential setting accordingly.

Having a child who presents with feeding issues can be a significant source of stress to parents or caregivers. It's inevitable that parents who themselves may be tired from a long day, when faced with the prospect of cooking a family meal and seeing at least one of the family completely bypass the presented meal on multiple occasions, are probably going to be reactive to such behaviour. Not only seen as a waste of time and effort but also a waste of money, it can be difficult to manage the prospect of a child going without nutrition. It's all too easy to enter a pattern of behaviour reflective of anger and guilt when such issues become commonplace.

It's important to realise that children quite easily pick up on such behaviours and their cycles. Without, hopefully, coming across all 'mother knows best' it's also important to understand that children can be very reactive to such cycles of behaviour in much the same way that pain to GI issues for example, can become a learned response affecting eating patterns. There are some simple ways of getting around such issues. Primary among them: relax. Children with or without autism generally do not starve themselves. Yes, we're bombarded with messages about the importance of 5-a-day and lots of other food propaganda added to the fact that there is a question circling the mind of many parents: what will they eat? But put all this to the back of your mind and relax. When parents relax, children relax. When parents' behaviour is relaxed towards food, children's' behaviour often eventually follows a similar pattern and this includes in relation to having a messy table and floor at the end of mealtimes.

> Parent and child stress over eating patterns and behaviours can have an effect

Parents might also want to set the boundaries. Tell your child how great the food is. Tell them how it's nutritious. Tell them that you're all going to sit together and the food is going to be on the table for 30 minutes at a set time. Tell them after that 30 minutes (dining rarely takes longer than this) has expired the plates are going to be cleared and any excess food is destined either for leftovers tomorrow or for composting. Be clear and stick to your rules consistently. Where other forms of communication are also used such as social stories or picture boards, think about how these can be adapted to convey a similar message.

Praise is an often under-used instrument at the dinner table. Praise can be a powerful motivator and when used proportionally, can be a greater changer of behaviour. It might be something as simple as praising a child for eating a single mouthful of a newly introduced food. Or for clearing their plate; even for putting their knife and fork on the plate when their meal is finished. And it works but like everything, use it sparingly and only when something genuinely merits praise (see Figure 8.1).

'I asked you to stop banging your spoon. You did it straight away. Thank you'

'I loved the way you shared with your brother/sister just now'

'Thank you for remembering to ask to leave the table'

Figure 8.1 Positive and descriptive praise examples.

There are several other ideas to try at the table. Empowering children to become active eaters is often a good strategy. Where possible, bring the food to the table in separate bowls or dishes and let the child select what they want and how much they want. You might have to help with serving, particularly when dishes are hot or where a child presents with those motor issues, but let them be in control of what they eat and be seen to be in control. Don't also be afraid to let a child smell, touch or lick a food before trying. These are basic senses which can often be great precursor behaviours to starting a new food or feeding behaviour. Obviously where there is a more negative behaviour such as throwing food, let them know this is not appropriate or acceptable. If you need to, clear the food away from the table immediately.

> Empowering people over their eating habits and patterns can be useful

Rewards, as we've hinted at with the example of ABA and autism, are already used in some cases. When it comes to food or other rewards at mealtimes, we would generally suggest that they are to be used sparingly (see Figure 8.2). It is far too easy for a reward to become part of a routine where 'for the easy life' a child sees eating their greens as just a stepping stone to the 'main', often sugary, event.

Non-food rewards that focus around the family can be a helpful tool to use when introducing new tastes and foods:

Collect rewards towards buying a family game, for example.
Use charts for coloured stickers or to colour in.
Use small items (age-appropriate) in a lucky dip box as a reward.
Use bricks for a tower the family build to an agreed height.
Read an extra story together.
Go for an outing e.g. park or favourite place of interest.

Figure 8.2 Reward ideas.

Allied to the issue of rewards is the concept of goal-setting and how the dinner table can and is a motivating learning experience. Figure 8.3 describes some of the basic steps of goal-setting behaviour where small goals are set and built upon using peas as an example. At each stage praise should accompany any progression to a next stage.

Step 1:	Place a single pea on a separate plate next to their main meal plate. You could use a plate with a favourite design or character on it. If accepted, proceed to the next step.
Step 2:	Place a single pea on their main meal plate. If accepted, proceed to the next step.
Step 3:	Add further peas (one at a time) to their main meal plate. If accepted, proceed to the next step.
Step 4:	Prompt the child to touch the peas on their plate. If accepted, proceed to the next step.
Step 5:	Prompt the child to smell the peas on their plate. If accepted, proceed to the next step.
Step 6:	Prompt the child to lick the peas on their plate. If accepted, proceed to the next step.
Step 7:	Prompt the child to put a single pea into their mouth and spit it back out on to their plate. If accepted, proceed to the next step.
Step 8:	Prompt the child to put a single pea into their mouth chew it and swallow it. If accepted, start the process with a new food.

Figure 8.3 Goal-setting.

In deciding what should be the next food to introduce in this goal-setting scheme you also have an opportunity to include the child in the process. So for example, prepare a new item list of foods and ask the child to rate them according to which they would prefer to try next. You could even include it as part of a game.

Mindfulness and mindful eating

No we've not moved into the realms of mumbo-jumbo as we begin some short discussion on the concept of mindfulness – the self-regulation of attention to focus on immediate experience. It's just that there are a growing number of people and organisations that have started to talk about the ways and means mindfulness might be able to control/manage issues like anxiety and depressive symptoms which can manifest alongside autism.[241]

There are quite a few authors with autism, generally more 'able' autism, talking about mindfulness and how it is an important part of maintaining their quality of life and impacting on the symptoms of their autism. Some of them have talked about the more negative effects of rumination – thinking repetitively about something – and how tackling such an issue via mindfulness training can be a great source of help in self-managing elements of their condition.

With regards to eating and feeding behaviour, mindfulness has also found some interest. The combined principles of pacing feeding behaviour, paying quite detailed attention to each mouthful of food, its smell, taste and texture, even the sensation of swallowing food with appropriate pauses in between, have been suggested to be a route towards things like weight loss and improving healthy eating among other things. In view of some of the issues described in relation to autism, there is some potentially good reason to ask whether mindfulness training might aid in overcoming eating issues where present. Obviously not everyone might be a suitable candidate because of the intensity of instruction that may be required, but if it's used as part of an overall package of managing symptoms there seems little harm in trying.

> Mindfulness techniques might be of help to some

More tips

There are various other hints and tips to try and include both during and outside of mealtimes. Try to use activities which support desirable eating habits. Play games together with food outside of mealtimes to help the child/person become more comfortable around food. Explore the different textures of food in the arena of play; for example using dried lentils or jelly as part of any play activities. Be creative too; make collages with food items or use them as part of other arts and crafts. At the same time, try and use more language to include food items such as counting using foods as examples or singing songs about food.

Story-telling is an ideal vehicle through which to introduce the topic of food. Whether it be replacing already known characters or inventing new ones around food, there is plenty of scope to keep food a topic of important conversation. In this context, don't also be afraid to really go to town with their imagination. Inventing food characters with for example, special powers such as x-ray vision carrots or super-power peas is a great way to bring food into the discussions and introduce conversation on the health benefits of certain foods and why they are important for a healthy, balanced diet. Ask the child to invent their own food character names and reinforce those healthy options.

You've probably already realised that association is an important part of making food and mealtimes more acceptable to a person. Keeping mealtimes fun and enjoyable rather than being associated with friction or a chore is an important part of redressing the relationship with food.

For the practical, hands-on side of things, you might also consider encouraging the child/person to grow their own food. This could be a window box growing herbs (mint, parlsey, thyme) or smaller vegetables. through to something altogether more adventurous in the garden. Such an activity can be coupled with play and games or even a diary plotting the project with, of course, the end-point being the consumption of the produce.

Pica, teeth and eating disorders

There is good reason to think that in some cases of autism, the presence of an unusual relationship with food might overlap into something approaching a food phobia. Given that anxiety seems to be something quite regularly linked to autism, one has to accept that this complicated mixture of presented symptoms might potentially perpetuate something seemingly trivial into something a whole lot more serious. Where there is a suspicion that food phobia may be present, it may be worth talking with a professional as to the measures which could be used to reduce this issue. Food phobia also highlights how other issues might also have the propensity to impact on feeding behaviours, such as the example of **pica**.

Pica describes where a person has persistent and sometimes compulsive cravings for eating non-food items or material. It can involve lots of different material including dirt, paper, paint, clothing and sand. In some cases even less desirable material such as faeces and hair are consumed. Whilst instances of pica during typical development are not necessarily all that unusual, particularly where young infants are still finding their way around the world and all its sensations, pica over a more extended period can place a person at increased risk of choking or ingestion of foreign items called bezoars which may require some surgical or other medical intervention. Where this happens, one could perhaps see how such extreme experiences of pica might directly impact on subsequent eating and feeding behaviour.

> Pica – the eating of non-edible objects and materials can be present in autism

With autism in mind, pica has been mentioned as appearing alongside cases although there is little data on precisely how frequent the condition might be. Most of the reports have tended to discuss extreme cases illustrating how pica ended up bringing a person to surgery,[242] or how pica might have been contributory to issues like lead intoxication[243] or indeed the **parasitic** risks attached to pica[244] (this last report not specifically mentioning autism *per se*). Again, all factors which could, one way or another, impact on the issue of feeding behaviours.

Pica is also connected with another issue which can impact on feeding behaviours; that is the state of those very important tools used during mastication (chewing), our teeth. As much as we would love to think about pica as always involving something nice and soft to chew on, that's not always the case. Stones, rocks and hardened, more artificial materials, can have quite profound effects on teeth, subsequently influencing the dietary choices open to a person.

The subject of teeth and oral hygiene represents another quite under-appreciated area of autism research and practice given that it crosses quite a few issues outside of just food and eating behaviours. Issues with teeth such as the presence of tooth decay (caries) or issues with the maturation of our gnashers (think wisdom teeth) have all been talked about in relation to cases of autism. The jury is still to some degree out on whether autism predisposes a person to a greater frequency of dental hygiene issues but certainly for some, there is evidence of poorer dental outcomes in some cases.[245] Such issues are not helped by the potential health inequalities which can appear as a result of the 'uncooperative' nature of some dental patients with autism[246] in terms of regular dental examinations. We don't think we need to say much more about how the state of a person's teeth might affect their eating habits.

> Strong teeth and good oral hygiene are essential for healthy eating

One final issue to cover when talking about feeding issues and autism is that of another comorbidity issue: eating disorders. Binge eating, anorexia nervosa and bulimia constitute the most common eating disorders: all reflective of a chaotic attitude to food which manifests in a person's eating habits. Again reiterating our notion that autism is seemingly protective of nothing when it comes to comorbidity, there is an emerging evidence base to suggest some degree of cross-over when it comes to the cognitive styles noted in cases of autism and cases of eating disorders.[247] What this work suggests is that some of the core characteristics of autism, particularly 'attention to detail' might also be a core feature of cases of eating disorder. This relationship in itself perhaps hints that eating disorders may not be uncommon in cases of autism, and appropriate screening should be implemented in suspected cases.

Starting a GFCF diet

Assuming that we've convinced you that there is actually some evidence for the possible effectiveness of a GFCF diet for cases of autism,[190] you might be wondering how one goes about adopting such an intervention. First things first, make that all-important appointment with your child's medical physician and talk things through with them. We've already mentioned in the Introduction that a good medical doctor can help if you wish to trial a GFCF diet on yourself or for a person in your care with regards to testing for **coeliac disease** for example. Without turning you or your child into a pin cushion, there may be other things that a doctor might suggest testing for such as **iron (ferritin)** levels. We're going to come on the **vitamins** and minerals shortly so we won't go too far into the heavy chemistry at this point.

If you or your child has a pre-existing medical condition such as something like **diabetes** or another food-related issue, it's even more important that you have contact with a medical healthcare professional before any dietary intervention is started. It's not only about the foods which are going to change but also the lifestyle alterations that this can bring, perhaps altering the amount of food you eat or the time of day at which you eat which can potentially also have knock-on effects for things like medication patterns for example.

Acknowledging that different parts of the world have different healthcare models, there is also good reason to bring in someone who specialises in dietetics and nutrition as part of the planning team when the decision is

> Seek professional medical and dietetic support prior to the implementation of diet

made to adopt a GFCF diet. Occupational labels and descriptions are different in different parts of the world but ensuring that your dietitian or nutritionist is suitably qualified to offer dietetic advice is important. It's even better when you find someone who specialises and has experience in using such dietary implementations with autism in mind. At the same time, use the Internet to have a look at someone's dietetic credentials and ask them questions, lots of them, about their experience in this area. If they're genuine, they won't mind answering you.

Already in our introduction we've provided you with a rough description of what **gluten** and **casein** are, and what foods one might reasonably assume to either have or not have gluten or casein in them. On purpose, we've chosen not to list 'safe' or 'risky' foods simply because we could take up pages doing so. There are resources out there which you can turn to, although we stress the need for professional help when first implementing dietary change.

Planning is vital when it comes to implementing a GFCF diet, as one might expect. The collected research on such dietary intervention for autism makes no mention of the dietary change being anything other than a long-term continued commitment. Certainly at the start of the intervention, there is the requirement for quite a lot of commitment on the part of those putting the diet in place. Make a list of all the people that you or your child has contact with over the course of a typical week. School teachers, carers, clubs and societies, extended family members such as grandparents should all be included. Anywhere and any situation where your child is not with you and hence likely to come into contact with food should figure on that list. Draft a short letter or email to each of these people or their organisations telling them what you are intending to do with regards to the dietary change.

We suggested right at the beginning of this book that everyone is part scientist. When it comes to the implementation of a GFCF diet we're going to show you another example of the scientific credentials that you

> Treat the implementation of the GFCF diet as a limited experiment

never knew you had. The best way of doing that is when it comes to starting the diet and the observations you're going to make over the course of the intervention. So, think about a start date. Think about when the transition over to a GFCF diet is going to cause least disruption to you or your child's routine. The various holiday seasons or any important social or religious events are probably not great times to begin a GFCF diet. Neither is the day of their birthday and all that entails. Once you have agreed on a start date, stick to it and include it in that letter or email you're going to be sending out to everyone concerned.

The next part of that start date relates to your undertaking a time-limited experiment of a GFCF dietary intervention. What that means is that as well as a start date, you're also going to be defining an end-point too; indeed several end-points in some cases. By saying this we're not suggesting that diet is some sort of quick fix which only needs to be adopted for a short period of time to work. The evidence doesn't suggest this to be the case and bearing in mind all those speculations on how and why diet might be working, many of those processes are relying on active and continual dietary change to be in place. The reason for the time limit is so you and others around you can take stock and as objectively as possible ask whether diet did indeed make any difference. The evidence you have at that point will be your guide.

Timescales for the effects of GFCF diet to be noticed? The question of how long your time-limited experiment should be in place is not an easy one to answer and to some extent it depends on how you go about introducing the GFCF diet. Two approaches exist: (a) the implementation of a casein-free diet first which then gradually adapts to include a gluten-free diet or (b) going 'all in' with a GFCF diet from day one. We would generally be minded to suggest that option (a), looking at implementation of a casein-free diet first, followed by the gluten-free diet, is the preferred course of action. Not only does this give you the ability to assess individual components of the diet, but it also makes the dietary transition just a little easier for everyone concerned. If you're going with option (a) you'll be looking at a first end-point assessment somewhere in the region of 8 weeks post implementation of a casein-free diet as representing your first evaluation. We base the judgement of 8 weeks casein-free upon the results of the study by Lucarelli and colleagues.[183]

The timescale to be looked at with the gluten-free diet in mind is slightly more complicated based on the available literature. Our previous, very preliminary, trial of a gluten-free diet alone[184] reported some effects following 5 months of intervention (approximately 20 weeks). The **ScanBrit trial** we dis-

> A suggested timescale: 8 weeks on casein-free diet 24 weeks on gluten-free diet

cussed earlier[180] talked about 8 months (32 weeks) of intervention before recording group changes to behavioural measures, bearing in mind this was a study of the combined GFCF diet. A timescale of 6 months (24 weeks) on a gluten-free diet would therefore represent a reasonable assumption to make on the basis of the currently available evidence. So if you're going to follow both diets, you'd be looking at a plan of something like that shown in Figure 8.4.

The next question is: how do you measure any difference in behaviour over the dietary periods? Again, we've highlighted the paper by Whiteley and colleagues[190] and the

Week 1: Start of diet (baseline). Introduction of a casein-free diet.   **Week 9**: Person on casein-free diet for 8 weeks.
Questions: Has it made a difference to behaviour or other aspects of daily functioning?   Do any positive changes noted merit continuation of the casein-free diet?
Week 10: Start of diet (baseline). Introduction of a gluten-free diet.   **Week 34**: Person on a gluten-free diet for 24 weeks.
Questions: Has it made a difference to behaviour or other aspects of daily functioning?   Do any positive changes noted merit continuation of the gluten-free diet (or combined diet if still following a casein-free diet too)?

Figure 8.4 A suggested timescale for GFCF dietary intervention.

summary of what types of changes have been reported from the various intervention studies. It used to be that the questionnaires and interviews were the tools of choice when it came to assess change in behaviour for whatever reason, but with the onset of the digital age, all of that has been superseded by our world being filmed and the wide availability of digital cameras. The good thing about such cameras is that nearly everyone has one and, particularly where parents and children are concerned, everyone's lives are to some extent documented these days.

Exactly what you film in relation to measuring dietary efficacy or not will to some extent depend on factors such as how old the child/adult is undertaking dietary intervention. You could go very science-like and set up a series of before and after challenges on which to record performance pre- and post-dietary intervention. Indeed, one of the gold-standard assessment schedules used for autism – the **Autism Diagnostic Observation Schedule (ADOS)**[248] – relies on just this situation to assess for the presence of autistic behaviours: recording the person's response to their name, asking them to play with some of their favourite toys and tell you what they're doing, smiling at them to see if they reciprocate, seeing if they use gestures like pointing, even asking them to write out a story or copy a piece of a story from a book, etc. With verbal children/adults, it's also useful to ask them about how they feel, what they think about their food pre- and post-dietary intervention and, indeed, whether they felt dietary intervention has made a change for the worse or better in their lives.

'Be scientific' when assessing the impact of dietary intervention

That all being said, it's not going to be possible to assess and video every aspect of a person's behaviour in the same way in such an objective fashion over the course of dietary intervention. Assessing whether hyperactive or impulsive behaviours are modified by the dietary change is not something easily documented, given their responsivity across different situations and under

Ask the person on diet whether they feel it has made a positive difference to them or not different conditions. Similarly, any changes to self-injurious behaviours or more physical issues like bowel problems are probably best logged the old-fashioned way on a frequency chart rather than filming events.

But even under such circumstances, there are ways to add an additional voice to that of parental opinion. It's always invaluable to ask whether others with a connection to the person can also contribute to evaluating diet over your experimental period. Teachers, for example, are ideally placed to provide their professional opinion on any change associated with the dietary period as a function of their role in observing and grading student progress in the classroom. Don't be afraid to ask them for their help.

Having then accumulated what is likely to be quite a lot of information on a person over the course of the dietary intervention period, the time then comes to ask the question: was it all worth it? In many respects this can be the most difficult part of the intervention. Often, there is a large degree of physical and emotional investment into getting the diet in place and maintaining it, alongside all the changes which it inevitably brings to family life. The psychological mantra of 'doing something' about the presentation of symptoms is ever-present and, for some parents, can itself be a significant source of comfort particularly where others roundabout might also be vocal about the use and effects of dietary intervention. But this is the time to weigh up the evidence in front of you. Have you seen a marked change in behaviour? Have others noticed a similar change? Do you feel that the person on diet is happier and has an improved quality of life as a result? Have some of the more disabling effects of autism or its comorbidities been reduced?

Although probably not great reading, for some people the answer to those questions is probably going to be no: over half a year spent following the experimental guidance we've offered and very little to show for it. Indeed like many other interventions, it's not necessarily a case of best effects vs. no effects, but rather best effects vs. worst effects as the person on a GFCF diet might have been further socially excluded as a result of their special dietary measures. It's not what people really want to hear but without any consistent criteria yet to gauge response other than trying diet, it's a scenario that readers need to be aware of.

> If diet didn't work, be honest and don't just continue for the sake of it

At this point it might also be useful for us to introduce the concept of ethics with regard to dietary change and autism. Ethics in this sense concerns the questions which have been raised about the rights and wrongs of interventions like the GFCF diet being implemented. Autism can be a minefield for ethics irrespective of what intervention is used. In cases where a person cannot give consent, informed consent, about various fundamental changes being implemented on their day-to-day lives, it means that to, a large extent, parents and professionals are reliant on the available evidence as indicating possible positive change and improvement in quality of life and are acting on that person's behalf and in their best interests. The big problem is that the evidence base is not by any means certain about lots of interventions used for autism, and indeed their potential real-world effects and side-effects outside of just their scientific study. It's been mentioned on more than one occasion that the implementation of a GFCF diet might itself raise certain ethical issues. Food as we've tried to illustrate is a tricky area for some people on the autism spectrum and following the implementation of an even more restrictive diet, which can often exclude quite a few of those 'staple foods', one can see how to some this could present problems. There are no easy answers to such ethical issues.

Core or peripheral effects?

We concluded Chapter 7, which looks at the proposed mode(s) of action of a GFCF diet, with a question on whether dietary intervention affects the core features of autism or rather impacts on more peripheral signs and symptoms. It's not a simple question to answer given that we still seemingly know so little about autism and its origins so can't readily assume what is being affected by something like a dietary change.

From the point of view of all those studies looking at gut permeability, gut bacteria, **enzymes** etc. one assumes that diet is having a secondary mechanistic effect on important centres such as the brain over and above directly affecting neurochemistry for example. So unlike the various behavioural and educational interventions which must be acting either structurally or chemically on the developing brain via their learning basis, the action of dietary change is less direct.

That being said, there is evidence from conditions like **schizophrenia** that where psychiatric symptoms present alongside organic diseases like coeliac disease, installation of a dietary change may have some considerable ability to affect various brain-imaging results. Take for example the results reported by De Santis and colleagues[249] illustrating how treatment of coeliac disease resolved behavioural symptoms and also positively affected blood flow to a specific part of the brain in their patient. The issue with autism is that no-one is yet looking at how diet affects brain imaging and scanning results.

> The question of whether the GFCF diet affects core or peripheral features is still largely unanswered

In terms of the proposed effects of diet on behaviour, the evidence so far seems to suggest that a mixture of both core and peripheral symptoms seem to be affected by the GFCF diet. The questions of what symptoms are affected first and whether this has knock-on effects for the presentation of other characteristics are unanswered. There are clues however to suggest that it's going to be a combination of issues being impacted by dietary intervention and these might not be the same for everyone. Drawing for example on the results reported by the ScanBrit trial,[180] one gets the impression that peripheral symptoms feature heavily in any dietary effect. So the results talking about group changes to inattention and hyperactivity are potentially going to impact on several important aspects of behaviour. Although still the topic of some speculation, changes to non-behavioural symptoms also discussed in relation to the GFCF diet such as bowel function are probably also going to impact on overall quality of life. In short it's not as easy as just quoting dietary effects on this or that function outside of the bigger picture of comorbidity and add-ons.

Vitamins and minerals

We've already touched on the issue of how looking at intake and levels of various vitamins and minerals might be an important issue to consider when looking at the possible usefulness of a GFCF diet. Defined as essential nutrients that the body needs to perform many of its vital duties in maintaining health and wellbeing, vitamins and minerals come in many different forms and have various uses.

In modern times we've all frankly become obsessed with how vitamins and minerals do this, that and the other. For some people, self-medication with vitamins and minerals is the drug of choice (yes, they are medicines) as we all aspire to increase our disease-free years and add vitality to our lives.

With autism in mind, there are literally hundreds of research findings covering nearly every aspect of vitamins and minerals far beyond the scope of this book. The theme in many cases is generally one of inadequate supplies of this or that **vitamin**, and how such deficiency can have serious knock-on effects for all manner of physiological processes including potential risk of autism as seen in all those **folic acid** discussions.[20] Indeed, by suggesting that a vitamin deficiency is present, for example, we immediately assign a value to how physiology is a part of autism, and based on some of the evidence so far, how correction of such vitamin deficiencies may very well impact on either risk of autism or the behavioural presentation of the condition.

Readers might already have noted from our discussion so far one reason why vitamin and/or mineral levels may be disrupted in cases of autism as a function of some of the GI issues we've talked about. Coeliac disease for example, has a long relationship with nutritional deficiency as a function of the malabsorption which goes hand-in-hand with symptoms. Outside of comorbidity with coeliac disease, the discussions in autism on gut permeability issues and various gut bacteria, some of which are able to manufacture nutrients, imply that similar issues might also be present.

Prof. Jim Adams, another parent turned autism researcher, has undertaken quite a lot of research looking at vitamins and minerals in relation to cases of autism. Perhaps one of his most important contributions to this area of research was the publication of his gold-standard trial of a vitamin and mineral supplement suggesting both nutritional and behavioural gains to be associated with its use on children with autism.[250] This follows on from earlier suggestions by another autism research pioneer, the late Dr Bernard Rimland, and his observations on **vitamin B6**.[251]

Specifically with the GFCF diet in mind, one could see how removal of foods containing gluten and **casein** from the diet might quite seriously impact on nutrient intake derived from these foodstuffs. Cereal products as well as being variously fortified are a good source of some of the B vitamins. Dairy products are synonymous with **calcium**. Both classes of vitamins/minerals are vital for growth and various essential biological processes throughout the body.

Calcium and vitamin D

One of the oft-cited questions heard when a casein-free diet is discussed in relation to autism is: 'but where will they get their calcium from?' You might be surprised to hear it from us but animal milk is a great food. It's crammed full of vitamins, minerals and fats and could almost be considered a meal in itself. There's good reason that at our earliest points in life, nature has supplied us with a meal from our mothers which does just about everything in terms of nutrition and so much more. At some point in human history, our ancestors decided that mother's milk was such a good resource that it would seek out similar alternatives. It did, and our worldwide consumption of animal milk from cows, goats, sheep and other mammals continues at a pace today.

One of the primary nutrients associated with milk is calcium. Calcium is a mineral; probably the most abundant mineral found in the body. Most of the calcium in the body is locked in bone and teeth where it performs a vital structural role although there are lots of other important duties given to calcium including the process of calcium signalling and other complicated biological actions taking place in our cells.

We've already talked about the downside for some people when drinking milk and how lactose intolerance or food protein intolerance syndromes like **FPIES** can be a feature of some cases of autism. The repercussions of removing milk and other dairy products from the diet have long been suspected to impact on calcium intake and, in cases of autism, the data suggest similar things can happen potentially impacting on important functions like bone health.[252] Indeed one of the main risks of a low calcium diet is the development of a condition called osteoporosis where bones thin and the risk of bones fractures in places like the wrist or hips is potentially increased.

The study by Hediger and colleagues[252] reporting on reduced bone cortical thickness in cases of autism and specifically those following a casein-free diet has been used almost hammer-like on occasions to stress how dangerous a GFCF diet can be. The results are important and certainly we would not stress otherwise, but set among a wider research context, they don't necessarily tell the whole story.

The study by Neumeyer and colleagues[253] likewise indicated that children with autism were more likely to present with bone issues, on the basis of their results looking at bone mineral density. Importantly, they also measured levels of circulating calcium and other parameters for their group, some of whom were following a GFCF diet. Moreover their findings of reduced bone mineral density found calcium levels to be equivalent between their autism and control groups, if anything, a little higher in their participants with autism. What they did suggest, however, was that physical activity levels were lower in their autism group and that levels of another important vitamin, **vitamin D,** were also lower in that group compared with control values.

Putting activity levels to one side, the findings of lower levels of vitamin D in cases of autism is a point of growing interest these days. Vitamin D can be made by the body following exposure to sunlight; hence its title 'the sunshine vitamin'. Derived from **cholesterol** – that stuff which has often wrongly gained the very worst reputation in modern medicine – vitamin D has lots of uses around the body including those related to proper immune function and brain development. There's even been a suggestion that vitamin D levels might also impact on gut permeability,[254] albeit with the requirement for further investigations. It is with calcium however that vitamin D has found its important partnership, and specifically how vitamin D aids in the absorption of calcium.

> Vitamin D is required to aid the proper absorption of calcium

Again with autism in mind, the results generally point towards a deficiency of vitamin D.[255] The results by Mostafa[255] are all the more interesting as a result of them being based on children with autism living in the Middle East, where unlike other parts of the world, sunshine is not normally in short supply. Interestingly the Hediger group have also noted similar instances of vitamin D deficiency in their subsequent studies.[256] In addition, other case studies report that known consequences of vitamin D deficiency such as rickets are also present in some children with autism.[257]

Whilst we are by no means trying to downplay the important role that calcium has or the fact that milk is a good source of calcium, set against the issue of vitamin D, one shouldn't automatically assume that a casein-free diet is a road to deficiency assuming that other foods or supplementation of both calcium and vitamin D are used as alternatives. Indeed where vitamin D deficiency is noted one could argue strongly that supplementation may be indicated and onwards speculate about any additional effects this might relate to.

Going back to the issue of calcium intake on a casein-free diet, there are several other foods which can help support calcium intake. Many of the alternative milks such as soya milk contain added calcium. Foods such as green leafy vegetables especially cooked spinach contain calcium as do dried fruits such as figs and apricots. Tinned sardines and salmon also contain calcium as a function of the small bones often consumed when eating these fish. One has to be mindful that these products generally do not contain as much calcium as milk (or not in a 'bioavailable' form) so more might need to be consumed to compensate for dairy removal from the diet.

The B vitamins (or vitamin B6 and vitamin B12 at least)

Excluding gluten from the diet does mean that the intake of certain nutrients might be reduced particularly some of the B vitamins. These vitamins are required for a diverse range of biological functions including energy release and growth. Whilst some gluten-free alternative products might be enriched with additional B vitamins, this sometimes does not altogether compensate for the loss seen when not eating gluten-containing cereal grains. Alternative sources of some of the B vitamins can be found in flaxseeds and other pulses and animal meat sources.

To talk about the B vitamins with autism in mind could potentially cover a lot of ground so we're going to have to be a little bit selective here and focus on two of the more studied ones: vitamin B6 and vitamin B12.

Vitamin B6, otherwise known as pyridoxine, has already been introduced by way of some of the discussions on the use of the vitamin in cases of autism normally in combination with the mineral magnesium. The story behind vitamin B6 and autism is not exactly clear but again it seems to have come out of various anecdotal reports from parents who observed changes to their child's behaviour following supplementation with so-called megadoses. The co-supplementation of magnesium seems to be due partly because of some proposed synergistic action, but also to negate some of the side-effects reported following vitamin B6 supplementation. Further scientific studies are warranted as to whether megadose vitamin B6 and magnesium should be generally indicated for autism.[258]

Quite a lot of the importance of vitamin B6 to autism lies in what form of the vitamin is present and whether the body can use it. Jim Adams (again) reported on higher levels of vitamin B6 detected in a group of children with autism compared with controls.[259] Importantly, he suggested that most of this vitamin load reflected the form of the vitamin which the body does not use, potentially indicative of issues with the conversion of the vitamin to the active, useable form – **pyridoxal 5 phosphate (PLP)** – in cases of autism.

> The active form of vitamin B6 is an essential part of making the neurotransmitter GABA

One of the important reactions which PLP is involved with is in the conversion of the excitatory neurotransmitter **glutamate** to the more inhibitory neurotransmitter **GABA** (gamma-Aminobutyric acid), where PLP aids the **enzyme** involved in this process. Glutamate and GABA have long been potential targets for autism research and specifically the design of various medicines to reduce the effects of glutamate and further support GABA function.

Vitamin B12 also has some history where autism is concerned. Vitamin B12, also called cobalamin, again represents several different compounds called vitamers. Going back to our discussions on regression and autism and that most interesting of diagnoses, Heller's syndrome or **CDD**, there

> Vitamin B12 deficiency has been associated with various behavioural effects

has been a suggestion that vitamin B12 deficiency may play an important role in some cases.[260] This is suggested to be part of a wider effect that vitamin B12 deficiency has been linked with.[261] There are quite a few angles from which issues with vitamin B12 have been tied into cases of autism. Our mention of some of the heated debate on a role for GI factors in cases of autism harks back to the now retracted paper by Wakefield and colleagues which suggested that levels of urinary **methylmalonic acid (MMA)** were elevated in cases of autism. Though the findings require replication, MMA has been suggested as a marker for vitamin B12 deficiency.[262] Supplementation with vitamin B12 or specifically methylcobalamin shows some potential for some people with autism although not seemingly for everyone.[263]

Iron

Of all the nutrients talked about with autism in mind, the mineral iron has perhaps been discussed the most.[264] Probably due to the relationship between iron and conditions like anaemia (iron-deficiency anaemia) and the adverse effects this can have on the developing child including providing an explanation for pica, iron is of some interest to autism research. Like the other vitamins and minerals already discussed, iron has some important biological effects in the body, such that any deficiency could potentially have far-reaching effects. Given also the various anecdotal reports of children with autism drinking sometimes quite a lot of milk and the subsequent negative impact of calcium on iron absorption, there is perhaps good reason to screen for iron deficiency in cases.

Iron levels can also change when a GFCF diet is initiated. Once again, green leafy vegetables can be a good source of iron (and fibre) bearing in mind that the plant origin of iron might also mean that the body requires more vitamin C to make the most of the available iron. Combining broccoli and peppers would, for example, be a good source of iron and vitamin C if included in something like a stir-fry. Eggs, beans and dried fruits also contain iron, and red meat and offal products such as liver are equally good for maintaining good iron levels.

Fibre

Whilst it's not a vitamin or mineral, it is important that we mention fibre (or fiber) in relation to the implementation of a GFCF diet. Fibre represents the part of our diet which passes through the body without generally being absorbed. Various cereal grains are high in fibre and hence related to the important function of keeping the gut healthy and bowel movements regular.

As one might expect, the removal of grains which contain gluten as part of the gluten-free diet may very well have some influence on the amount of fibre contained in the diet and, as a result, on bowel function. Thinking back to our earlier discussions on the various functional bowel issues that have been reported in relation to autism, one could therefore envisage a scenario where a reduction in dietary fibre might exacerbate such problems.

Nevertheless, there are various gluten-free grains which can aid in increasing fibre intake on a GFCF diet. Brown rice, amaranth, buckwheat and quinoa are all useful additions to the diet as a function of their fibre content. Corn, even popcorn, can be used to increase fibre content; although please be sparing with the salt or sugar if you choose to flavour popcorn.

You're gonna need a bigger boat

Acknowledging that there is a lot to take in from this chapter, we've hopefully provided you with a few pointers about the practicalities of undertaking a GFCF diet. We've tried to stress how, irrespective of the word 'diet' and any opinions this carries about the approach, there is good reason to treat the GFCF option the same you would any other intervention for autism and be meticulous in its planning and execution. This includes fostering your inner scientist to try, as far as possible, to objectively test the diet in a time-limited fashion and bringing in appropriate medical and dietetic help accordingly. Given the often significant issues with food which can accompany a diagnosis with autism, it's even more imperative that this dietary approach is not entered into lightly for the sake of you and your family but most importantly, to benefit the person on whom the diet is being thrust.

Foods which contain gluten and casein are everywhere and as we've discussed, even these 'bad guys' carry lots of potential nutritional benefits which, when a person is on the GFCF diet, will need to be derived from other sources. Most people who have cleared the introduction of diet and found it to have effects worthy of its continuation do become pretty expert on what can and can't be eaten on the diet. In some cases, the GFCF diet morphs into other dietary interventions; although we offer no opinion on this course of action. All we would stress is that continual monitoring be in place to watch out for things like nutritional deficiency and importantly, how quality of life might change as a result of a person getting older and perhaps having more of a say in how their life is led.

In the final chapter (yes, you're almost there), we're going to talk about a few of the other important findings which encircle the GFCF diet applied to autism. We're not going to try and relate everything back to diet and autism but we will provide food for thought on how some previously discussed elements might relate to one another.

References

233. Barnevik Olsson M. *et al.* Autism before diagnosis: crying, feeding and sleeping problems in the first two years of life. *Acta Paediatr.* 2013; 102: 635–639.
234. Whiteley P. Developmental, behavioural and somatic factors in pervasive developmental disorders: preliminary analysis. *Child Care Health Dev.* 2004; 30: 5–11.
235. Whiteley P. *et al.* Feeding patterns in autism. *Autism.* 2000; 4: 207–211.
236. Jarocka-Cyrta E. *et al.* Eosinophilic esophagitis as a cause of feeding problems in autistic boy. The first reported case. *J Autism Dev Disord.* 2011; 41: 372–374.
237. Buie T. *et al.* Recommendations for evaluation and treatment of common gastrointestinal problems in children with ASDs. *Pediatrics.* 2010; 125 Suppl 1: S19–S29.
238. Ibrahim SH. *et al.* Incidence of gastrointestinal symptoms in children with autism: a population-based study. *Pediatrics.* 2009; 124: 680–686.
239. Stewart ME. *et al.* Presentation of depression in autism and Asperger syndrome: a review. *Autism.* 2006; 10: 103–116.
240. Betalli P. *et al.* Autism and esophageal achalasia in childhood: a possible correlation? Report on three cases. *Dis Esophagus.* 2013; 26: 237–240.
241. Spek AA. *et al.* Mindfulness-based therapy in adults with an autism spectrum disorder: a randomized controlled trial. *Res Dev Disabil.* 2013; 34: 246–253.
242. Serour F. *et al.* Intestinal obstruction in an autistic adolescent. *Pediatr Emerg Care.* 2008; 24: 688–690.
243. Shannon M. & Graef JW. Lead intoxication in children with pervasive developmental disorders. *J Toxicol Clin Toxicol.* 1996; 34: 177–181.

244. Mumtaz S. *et al.* Frequency and risk factors for intestinal parasitic infection in children under five years age at a tertiary care hospital in Karachi. *J Pak Med Assoc.* 2009; 59: 216–219.

245. Jaber MA. Dental caries experience, oral health status and treatment needs of dental patients with autism. *J Appl Oral Sci.* 201; 19: 212–217.

246. Loo CY. *et al.* The caries experience and behaviour of dental patients with autism spectrum disorder. *J Am Dent Assoc.* 2008; 139: 1518–1524.

247. Coombs E. *et al.* An investigation into the relationship between eating disorder psychopathology and autistic symptomatology in a non-clinical sample. *Br J Clin Psychol.* 2011; 50: 326–338.

248. Lord C. *et al.* Autism diagnostic observation schedule: a standardized observation of communicative and social behavior. *J Autism Dev Disord.* 1989; 19: 185–212.

249. De Santis. *et al.* Schizophrenic symptoms and SPECT abnormalities in a coeliac patient: regression after a gluten-free diet. *Journal Intern Med.* 1997; 242: 421–423.

250. Adams JB. *et al.* Effect of a vitamin/mineral supplement on children and adults with autism. *BMC Pediatr.* 2011; 11: 111.

251. Rimland B. *et al.* The effect of high doses of vitamin B6 on autistic children: a double-blind crossover study. *Am J Psychiatry.* 1978; 135: 472–475.

252. Hediger ML. *et al.* Reduced bone cortical thickness in boys with autism or autism spectrum disorder. *J Autism Dev Disord.* 2008; 38: 848–856.

253. Neumeyer AM. *et al.* Bone density in peripubertal boys with autism spectrum disorders. *J Autism Dev Disord.* 2012 Nov 4.

254. Kong J. *et al.* Novel role of the vitamin D receptor in maintaining the integrity of the intestinal mucosal barrier. *Am J Physiol Gastrointest Liver Physiol* 2008; 294: G208–G216.

255. Mostafa G. & Al-Ayadhi LY. Reduced serum concentrations of 25-hydroxy vitamin D in children with autism: relation to autoimmunity. *J Neuroinflammation.* 2012; 9. 201.

256. Molloy C. *et al.* Plasma 25(OH)D concentration in children with autism spectrum disorder. *Dev Med Child Neurol.* 2010; 52: 969–971.

257. Stewart C. & Latif A. Symptomatic nutritional rickets in a teenager with autistic spectrum disorder. *Child Care Health Dev.* 2008; 34: 276–278.

258. Nye C. & Brice A. Combined vitamin B6-magnesium treatment in autism spectrum disorder. *Cochrane Database Syst Rev* 2005; 4: CD003497.

259. Adams JB. *et al.* Abnormally high plasma levels of vitamin B6 in children with autism not taking supplements compared to controls not taking supplements. *J Altern Complement Med.* 2006; 12: 59–63.

260. Malhotra S. *et al.* Brief Report: Childhood Disintegrative Disorder as a likely manifestation of vitamin B12 deficiency. *J Autism Dev Disord.* 2013 Jan 20.

261. Dror DK. & Allen LH. Effect of vitamin B12 deficiency on neurodevelopment in infants: current knowledge and possible mechanisms. *Nutr Rev.* 2008; 66: 250–255.

262. Yetley EA. *et al.* Biomarkers of vitamin B-12 status in NHANES: a roundtable summary. *Am J Clin Nutr.* 2011; 94: 313S–321S.

263. James SJ. *et al.* Efficacy of methylcobalamin and folinic acid treatment on glutathione redox status in children with autism. *Am J Clin Nutr.* 2009; 89: 425–430.

264. Reynolds A. *et al.* Iron status in children with autism spectrum disorder. *Pediatrics.* 2012; 130 Suppl 2: S154–S159.

RECIPES

Peppers stuffed with amaranth and chorizo

A perfect light lunch that can be made in advance (serves 4).

Ingredients

4 red peppers
100 grams of amaranth or rice
1/2 stock cube
Water
100 grams of chorizo, finely diced
1 dessertspoon of rapeseed oil
1 large red onion
1 carrot
3 cloves of garlic (or to taste)
1 tablespoon of tomato paste

Method

Preheat an oven to 180 degrees centigrade/gas mark 4. Fill and boil a kettle full of water. Chop the peppers in half lengthways, remove the core and seeds, place on a baking tray and bake in the oven for 20 minutes. Add the amaranth or rice and stock cube to a pan of water, bring to the boil and then allow to simmer for 20 minutes. Finely chop the chorizo, add to a medium pan on a medium heat and allow to cook for 5 minutes. Peel and finely chop the onion and carrot and add to a medium pan with the oil. Cook gently until the onion is turning translucent after about 5 minutes. Crush the garlic and add to the onion mixture and cook for a further minute. Add the chorizo and tomato paste and cook the tomato paste for a minute. Add the amaranth and stir to combine. Remove the peppers from the oven and fill with the mix.

Sprinkling of nutritional science

Naturally gluten- and casein-free, amaranth grain is a great alternative to other grains used in cooking. A great source of magnesium, phosphorus and **vitamin B6** when cooked, amaranth grain was enjoyed and revered by the ancient Aztecs and still finds some popularity across the globe. Consumption of amaranth grain, a good source of fibre, is thought to confer various health-related properties not least in lowering cholesterol and potentially affecting the production of chemicals related to **allergy**.

Chestnut and mushroom loaf

A vegetarian alterative to the traditional meat loaf, ideal for freezing (serves 8–12).

Ingredients

25 grams of dairy-free margarine
1 small onion, peeled and finely chopped

1 large clove garlic, finely sliced
2 sticks of celery, finely chopped
150 grams of finely chopped chestnut mushrooms (you can use other varieties also)
400 grams of chestnuts (fresh★ or vacuum packed), chopped
200 grams of cashew nuts, chopped
1 tablespoon of gluten-free flour
100 millilitres of Madeira (you can also use red wine but Madeira gives a better flavour)
1 egg, beaten
1 tablespoon of Tamari soy sauce
2 tablespoons of chopped parsley
¼–½ teaspoon of smoked paprika (depending on how much heat you wish)

Method

Preheat the oven to 200 degrees centigrade. You may find it easier to use a food processor to help with the chopping. To a large heavy based pan add the dairy-free margarine, add the onion and sauté for 2 minutes. Add the garlic, celery and mushrooms and cook gently for 3–4 minutes. Add the flour and Madeira and mix through until the mixture thickens. Add the rest of the ingredients mix so it's all evenly distributed. Pack into a greased loaf tin, cover with foil, place in a bain-marie and bake in the oven for 1 hour. A bain-marie is a deep tray filled part way with water; the level of the water should be below the loaf tin about 3/4 way up. Lift out and allow to cool. Slice into portions. Slices can be frozen to use at a later date. Serve in place of meat on a roast dinner with an onion gravy.

★ To cook fresh chestnuts, use a sharp knife to cut a cross into the skin on the flattest side, place in a pan of water and cook for 15 minutes, allow to cool, then peel off the skins.

Sprinkling of nutritional science

Harvested from the cashew tree and in particular from the cashew apple, cashew nuts are a great addition to many dishes. As with many other nuts, their health benefits stem from their oil content – principally unsaturated fats – and their generous mineral content. A good source of zinc and iron, cashew nuts also provide a plentiful supply of trace minerals such as copper and magnesium, essential elements for various enzymes functioning throughout the body.

Lamb tagine

A taste of Morocco is only a pan away (serves 4).

Ingredients

1 teaspoon of cayenne pepper
2 teaspoons of ground black pepper
1½ tablespoons of paprika
1½ tablespoons of ground ginger
1 tablespoon of turmeric
2 teaspoons of ground cinnamon

1 tablespoon of smoked paprika
1 shoulder of lamb, trimmed and cut into 5cm / 2 inch chunks (about 1kg of meat in total)
2 large onions, finely chopped
2 tablespoons of rapeseed or olive oil
3 cloves garlic, crushed
2 x 400g tinned chopped tomatoes
115 grams of dried apricots, cut in half
55 grams of dates, chopped
100 grams of flaked almonds
600 millilitres of gluten-free lamb stock or chicken stock or add some homemade bouillon water
1 tablespoon of clear honey
2 tablespoon of flat leaf parsley, roughly chopped to garnish

Method

Place the cayenne, black pepper, paprika, ginger, turmeric and cinnamon into a small bowl and mix together. Place the lamb in a large bowl and toss together with the spice mix. Cover and leave overnight in the fridge. Preheat the oven to 150 degrees centigrade / gas mark 2. Heat 1 tablespoon of olive oil in a large casserole dish. Add the onions and cook over a gentle heat for 10 minutes so that the onions are soft but not coloured. Add the crushed garlic and cook for a further 3 minutes. In a separate frying pan, heat the remaining oil and brown the cubes of lamb on all sides then add the browned meat to the casserole dish. De-glaze the frying pan with some of the tomato juice and add these juices to the pan. Add the remaining tomato juice, stock, chopped tomatoes, apricots, dates, flaked almonds, lamb stock and honey to the casserole dish. Bring to the boil, cover with a fitted lid, place in the oven and cook for 2–2½ hours or until the meat is meltingly tender. Place the lamb in a tagine or large serving dish and sprinkle the chopped herbs over it.

Sprinkling of nutritional science

A tasty accompaniment to meat dishes, parsley may also confer some important health benefits for some people. Whilst pregnant women are generally advised to limit their parsley intake, for others parsley is a good source of vitamin C and folic acid. Parsley also contains antioxidants including luteolin and apigenin which are thought to possess important anti-inflammatory and, potentially, anti-cancer properties.

Lime drizzle cake

Strange ingredients but try this zesty treat... delicious! (serves 8–12).

Ingredients

200 grams of dairy-free margarine
200 grams of caster sugar
4 eggs
175 grams of ground almonds
250 grams of mashed potato

Zest of 3 limes
2 tablespoons of gluten-free baking powder

For the drizzle
4 tablespoons of honey
Juice of 2 limes

Method

Heat the oven to 180 degrees centigrade / fan oven 160 degrees / gas mark 4. Coat and a deep 20cm diameter cake tin with a little of the margarine. Beat the sugar and margarine together until light and fluffy, and then gradually add the egg, beating after each addition. Fold in the almonds, cold mashed potato, lime zest and baking powder. Tip into the tin, level the top, then bake for 40–45 minutes or until golden brown when a skewer inserted into the middle of the cake comes out clean. Turn out on to a wire rack after 10 minutes cooling. Mix the honey and the lime juice together, then spoon over the top of the cake, letting it drip down the sides. Let the cake cool completely before slicing.

Sprinkling of nutritional science

Adorning many a plate of food or snack, the potato represents one of the staple foods of modern-day living. The science behind the potato is rather mixed as associations between chemicals such as solanine and acrylamide (following cooking at high temperatures) and their potentially negative effects on health continue to generate headlines. But don't put the humble potato out to pasture just yet as this starchy crop contains a host of important vitamins and minerals including, surprisingly, quite a high proportion of vitamin C.

Chapter 9

The broader picture

Having already covered quite a bit of the autism research environment with GFCF dietary intervention in mind, there are a few areas of interest which we also want to talk about in this book. As with many things connected to autism, it's often best not to view these findings as being stand-alone, but rather pieces of a giant puzzle which in some way, shape or form all fit together even though we might not currently have the tools or ability to see the complete picture. Food and diet in relation to autism feature in quite a lot of the discussions but we cover various other related areas too. Continue reading and humour us.

Other diets, other conditions

The overlap between the **schizophrenia** and autism spectrums is an area seeing a resurgence of research interest in recent years. On purpose we've included quite a bit of discussion on schizophrenia because of the realisation that there may be shared aetiological agents between the conditions. The interesting role of **gluten** and **casein** in cases of schizophrenia and autism also hints at some shared pathways and therapeutic targets. Indeed the suggestion that a **GFCF diet** might be a potential intervention option for autism stems to a large extent from the work of the late Curt Dohan and his observations of schizophrenia and food.[265]

Dietary intervention for schizophrenia is a growth research area

The continued interest in schizophrenia and gluten and casein has continued over the intervening years, to some extent overtaking what has been done in autism research circles. At the same time, however, such research in schizophrenia potentially provides valuable clues as to where autism research could also start looking. This includes the analysis of antibodies specifically to fractions of gluten such as gliadin[266] and the complement system,[267] similar analysis of antibodies to casein,[268] findings based on markers of GI **inflammation** such as anti-Saccharomyces cerevisiae **IgG antibodies (ASCA)**[269] and the possibility of **parasitic** infections also being involved in the way the immune system handles certain foods.[270] There is currently no suggestion that autism and schizophrenia will present with the same pattern of dietary issues under some unifying banner of food-related themes. But without the appropriate studies being carried out in autism, nor can one rule out any commonalities occurring.

A similar food-related theme has also been discussed with another important condition often comorbid to autism in mind: **ADHD**. Readers are perhaps starting to understand why we dedicated such a large chunk of this book to the add-ons which can quite often follow a diagnosis of autism. With ADHD in mind, food, or rather various elements of the diet, has been quite a persistent theme down the years as being linked to the presentation of symptoms. Initially greeted with a large degree of scepticism, more recently there has been an acknowledgment that certain features of the modern diet may very well have the ability to impact on the presence of ADHD or some of its core features.[271]

Outside of looking at food colourings and preservatives as potentially influencing some of the characteristics of ADHD following the suggestions of the **Feingold diet**,[272] other research has suggested some merit in looking at rotation diets in cases of ADHD.[273] Perhaps the most interesting thing about the diet looked at in the Pelsser study and other attempts[274] from the point of view of this book was the reduction in foods containing gluten and casein as a result of their installation of a hypoallergenic (not provoking an immune response) foods diet.

Again, there are perhaps lessons that autism research can learn from the literature looking at diet and ADHD. Of even greater interest than the body of work on diet and schizophrenia is the notion that the positive dietary effects being noted in cases of autism as a result of the institution of a GFCF diet tend to also include behaviours which fall into the ADHD domain such as inattention and hyperactivity. Whether this provides further evidence of a link between ADHD and autism and, indeed, the possibility of shared intervention pathways is still the source of speculation.

We've mentioned how the GFCF diet for autism represents probably the most popular dietary intervention currently in use and also carries the lion's share of research and opinion to boot. To say that the GFCF diet is the only dietary 'option' for autism would, however belittle the growing evidence base in various other diet-related areas, some of which are potentially overlapping.

> ADHD-type behaviours have been reported as a target for the GFCF diet in autism

Our discussions on the area of **carbohydrate** metabolism in relation to autism have already hinted at how there may be sound logic in further examination of diets limiting carbohydrate intake such as the **SCD** and **GAPS diet** in some cases. Of potential relevance to this area is the increasing interest in the use of a **ketogenic diet** for autism and, indeed, some of its important **comorbidity**. If you're wondering what a ketogenic diet is, think low carbohydrate and high fat intake. You'll probably know of something similar if you've heard of man called Robert Atkins and his contribution to the thriving weight loss industry.

With autism research in mind, the ketogenic diet is still a work in progress. The very preliminary results following experimental trial of the ketogenic diet in cases of autism by Evangaliou and colleagues[275] hinted at the possibility of some effect. This has been followed up by case studies[276] and work using mouse models.[277] The question of how exactly the ketogenic diet works in autism is still an unanswered one. A ketogenic diet by its very nature is designed to make the body switch fuel sources to burning fats rather than sugars, part and parcel of which involves the production of ketones and a state of ketosis. It is with this process in mind that the diet has, under experimental conditions, been noted to have some quite prominent effects on certain cases of **epilepsy**.[278] The case report by Herbert and Buckley[276] has offered a few reasons why, outside of just a reduced **carbohydrate** load, the ketogenic might impact on the presentation of autism. The subject of their case report presented with both autism and epilepsy. Following use of the ketogenic diet, she was after some months on dietary intervention categorised as 'essentially seizure

> The ketogenic diet – low carbs, high fat – has been proposed as an intervention for autism

free'. One might reasonably assume that by affecting seizure patterns and activity the diet might also have had a knock-on effect on mechanisms which affect presented behaviour. Certainly such a hypothesis makes for a strong research requirement to further monitor the effects of dietary change on the central nervous system in cases of autism and its various comorbidities.

There are several other dietary regimes which have been suggested for autism and some its comorbidities. To detail them all is beyond the scope of this book but we will in passing mention the very preliminary data put forward as evidence for the potential of a **low oxalate diet**[279] with the recommendation for much further study. We're not entirely done with diets and autism as you'll see in our subsequent discussions on the various inborn errors of metabolism in relation to the condition coming up. But for now we hope you can appreciate how to talk about diet and autism might not necessarily just mean talking about one thing.

Immune functions

We've mentioned autism and immune system a few times in this book already without any formal introduction about what the immune system is and what it does. 'Protection' is probably the most simple way of describing your immune system, and how without it we'd have all gone the way of the dodo a long time back.

Like many things about the human body, the immune system is a remarkable piece of equipment. Generally subdivided into the innate and adaptive immune systems, its crowning achievement is the ability to distinguish between the body or self, and thousands upon thousands of bacteria, viruses and other nasties (other) which want to either feast upon us or call us home (or both).

That's not, however, to say that the immune system always runs at peak efficiency. Inactivity of the immune system and its functions can trigger immunodeficiencies, whereby the body is not able to mount the response required to recognise and clear away pathogens. An overactivity of the immune system can lead to **autoimmunity**, whereby the immune system fails to recognise the body as self and so attacks part of it as if it were 'other'. If you think back to our discussions on **coeliac disease**, you've got a good example of how autoimmunity can manifest in the GI tract as a function of foods containing gluten. It's all about maintaining a balanced protective approach for the immune system.

> Numerous authors have discussed a possible role for the immune system in cases of autism

There is a huge expanse of research on the immune system and immune function with autism in mind: certainly far too vast for us to include even the main themes in such a short section in this book. So, we're going to run through only a small part of that work and in particular, those topics close to our dietary hearts. What we'll also say is that when it comes to the immune system and autism, there is no one-size-fits-all, almighty theory of how it works in autism. Indeed, to say it's complicated and often counter-intuitive is perhaps an understatement.

Maternal immune activation

Readers have already been introduced to the work of Paul Patterson and colleagues[19] looking at mouse models of immune activation potentially mapping on to cases of autism.

The theory is that maternal exposure to some infective agent during a period of pregnancy might have the ability to invoke certain lasting effects on the immune and behavioural functions of offspring which could manifest as autistic-like behaviours. At least in mice. Some of Prof. Patterson's most recent investigations[111] at the time of writing have further expanded that immune–behaviour link to suggest that issues like gut hyperpermeability (**leaky gut**) might also be a feature of offspring, treatable by use of a **probiotic**. Again at least in mice.

With our interest in diet and autism and some of the mechanisms we've discussed, readers can perhaps see how exciting this work is. Indeed, also introducing a new element into the gut–brain relationship to be rebranded as the gut–immune–brain relationship. The suggestion being that outside of just policing and protecting against infectious or other agents, the immune system and all its myriad of chemical and cocktails involved in processes like inflammation and autoimmunity might also have the ability to affect human behaviour and psychological development.

Let's just take a few steps back. There is some support for the notion of maternal immune activation being potentially linked to risk of autism outside of just mouse models. Examination of levels of markers of inflammation such as C-reactive protein in mothers who went on to have a child with autism has suggested a correlation.[280] Other reports of maternal fever during pregnancy being linked to offspring autism risk[281] complement the association made. Coupled with more direct observations of the immune system acting on behaviour potentially leading to autism through for example the action of **microglia**[282,283] there is evidence for a potential effect. Microglia – a part of the immune system resident in the brain – are of particular interest in their gardening role,[284] pruning parts of the brain during early development.

The other strand of work in this area revolves around the suggestion that the immune system of mothers who subsequently have a child with autism might be uniquely predisposed to attack certain brain protein of their children.[285] Whilst sounding all rather dramatic, there is a growing evidence base to this suggestion[286] including studies documenting the quite dramatic effects of injecting such brain antibodies taken from mothers into a mouse model.[287]

> Maternal immune activation during pregnancy is suggested to impact on offspring development

Autoimmunity and the hygiene hypothesis

Without going over previously trodden ground, coeliac disease, one of the archetypal autoimmune conditions, can and does appear in cases of autism. Indeed, according to the observations by Genuis,[91] treating coeliac disease with a gluten-free diet might also have the ability to impact on some of the features of autism in certain cases where it does coexist.

There are signs of an emerging relationship between autoimmunity and autism. One of the earliest papers to discuss the possibility that autoimmune conditions might encircle families with a person with autism came from Money and colleagues[288] in 1971. They described a 'rare phenomenon' of autism set amongst a family history of conditions like ulcerative colitis – yes, that bowel condition we talked about earlier – and other autoimmune conditions. Given the subsequent literature looking at autoimmunity in families where autism is present, we might question the notion that this is a rare occurrence. Ulcerative colitis, for example, has been reported to be more frequent in parents of children with autism, alongside other autoimmune conditions such as type-1 diabetes.[289]

One of the particularly interesting features of autoimmune conditions is that they tend to 'clump' together. So if you are diagnosed with type-1 diabetes, you're more likely to also present with coeliac disease[290] and likewise the relationship between other autoimmune conditions such as psoriasis or rheumatoid arthritis. What this and the familial association of autoimmunity and autism might imply is that either one factor can potentially affect the risk of the other, or even more speculatively, that autism, some autism, may in fact represent an autoimmune condition.[291]

> Autoimmunity has been reported to be a feature of some cases of autism

That last sentence, referenced we might add by a paper from researchers working at the MIND Institute in the USA, is quite provocative but not potentially absolutely wrong. We've already talked about **tissue transglutaminase (tTG)** and its frequency in cases of autism.[90] Other peripheral markers of autoimmunity such as IL-17 secreted by **Th17**cells have been discussed with autism in mind.[292] In layman's terms, Th17 – T helper 17 cells – represent a relatively new arm of the immune system thought to play a large role in the progression of various autoimmune and inflammatory conditions. They secrete various chemical messengers including compounds called **cytokines**, the currency of the immune system. IL-17 or more specifically IL-17A is one of those cytokines found by Al-Ayadhi[292] to be elevated in their participant group with autism.

One of the suggestions put forward to account for the seeming increasing in autoimmune conditions both in cases of autism and in the general population is the changing relationship we have with our environment and the notion of the hygiene hypothesis.[293] The hypothesis speculates that as our environment has got cleaner – our food nicely packaged up and free of bugs and stuff, our drinking water cleansed, our living conditions being a whole lot different from even a century or two back – so the relationship we have with microbes and viruses has changed. Most of that change has been one of depletion of our contact with such organisms, particularly during our early days. The net result is that immune system does not have the necessary contact with the baddies and so goes its own way. We might add that gut bacteria are also thought to play a role in this process.

It might all sound a million miles away from our discussions on the GFCF diet and autism, but there are some potentially relevant links to be noted. The opinion piece by Moses Velasquez-Manoff[294] summarised it all pretty well, uniting areas like the mouse model of maternal immune activation to gut bacteria to the prevalence of autoimmunity alongside cases of autism, with the immune system proposed to be an important feature in the presentation of autism and its effects indeed doing so much more than just fighting infection.

The amino acids and friends

Amino acids. Y'know those individual pearls of the **protein/peptide** necklace that we talked about in a previous chapter? Well, it turns out that outside of just being a vital source of nutrition it may be that they have much more influence on our health and wellbeing.

Phenylalanine and phenylketonuria (PKU)

We've already introduced one amino acid to you in relation to food and mental health: phenylalanine

> Phenylketonuria – PKU – is the archetypal 'diet can affect mental health' condition

and the inborn metabolic error of **phenylketonuria (PKU)**. Think about that drop of blood taken from the heel of most newborns and you already know something about PKU. The **Guthrie heel prick test** is used to look for the tell-tale signs of PKU, in particular a build-up of phenylalanine in the blood which can damage the brain. For those babies who show the signs of PKU the treatment is via a low protein diet and specifically the avoidance of phenylalanine, complemented by supplementation with another amino acid made from phenylalanine, tyrosine. It's little wonder then that PKU is known as the archetypal 'diet can affect behaviour' condition. Although the overall prevalence of PKU is low, it does have quite a classical connection with autism.[295]

One or two of the newer interventions proposed for PKU also have quite interesting connections to cases of autism. Get ready for a word to amaze your friends with: tetrahydrobiopterin. Also more conveniently known as **BH4**, tetrahydrobiopterin is a naturally occurring compound in the body. Similar to the action of one or two of the vitamins we've talked about, BH4 is used as a **cofactor** for quite a few important biological reactions in the body. One of those reactions just happens to be with phenylalanine in mind, and its conversion to tyrosine.

Autism has also been talked about with BH4 in mind. The investigations are still quite preliminary but outside of lower levels of BH4 noted in cases of autism[296] there is some suggestion that it might potentially be a therapeutic option.[297] As to the question of why BH4 might affect the presentation of autism, well, we've got our opinions on things like its ability to work as a cofactor for other enzymes which convert amino acids to neurotransmitters, but no-one really knows for sure.

The branched chain amino acids and carnitine

Working out the relative weighting of genetics and environment in terms of how they might elevate risk of autism and also provide clues as to the course of the condition has been a primary aim for many people for many years. With the advent of research looking at the possibility of other inborn errors of metabolism focused on amino acids presenting in cases of autism, there are some interesting pointers emerging for at least some of the autisms.

The paper by Gaia Novarino and colleagues[298] represented quite a leap in autism research circles. Again with amino acids in mind, specifically a family of amino acids called the **branched–chain amino acids**, Novarino reported on a genetic mutation as being present in some cases of autism comorbid to **intellectual disability** and epilepsy. The mutation hindered the processing of these branched–chain amino acids. More than that, however, were the initial results (in a mouse model of this mutation) which suggested that supplementation with amino acids like valine, leucine and isoleucine might abate some of the symptoms reported. Again, we aren't necessarily advocating dietary supplementation of branched–chain amino acids or anything at this point. But the results are promising and reiterate our very important relationship with food and its constituent components.

> Various conditions affecting amino acid chemistry have been linked to the presence of autism

We've also included mention of the compound **carnitine** in this section despite the fact that it isn't actually an amino acid. This amino acid pretender – made by an amino acid – actually covers a number of carnitines which have various important actions throughout the body. With autism in mind, carnitine has some history. Levels of carnitine have been reported to be lower in cases of autism and thought by some authors to tie into a **mitochondrial** defect.[299] Think back to our earlier discussions on the cell powerhouse for example.

It was, however, another important paper by Patrícia Celestino–Soper and colleagues[300] which fits into our discussions on inborn errors of metabolism potentially manifesting as autism. They reported genetic issues with the synthesis of carnitine and their prevalence in cases of autism. Also important was their suggestion that supplementation with carnitine may be a therapeutic option for some cases.

MTHFR and the big 'H'

Hopefully you're still with us as we explore one final group of amino acids and their potential importance to autism. The amino acids in question are all linked to one another and, in many respects, form one of the most obvious interactions between environment and genetics, or at least **epigenetics**.

First up is the amino acid **homocysteine** (the big 'H'). Homocysteine is generally another compound with quite a bad reputation. Its 'association' with various physical health complaints has been the topic of considerable discussion and debate. Homocysteine levels in cases of autism are generally described as being elevated; indeed quite consistently so.[301] The question of why elevated levels of homocysteine are present in autism and what their relevance might be is still under investigation.

As you might be able to see from Figure 9.1, of some importance is the link between homocysteine and another amino acid called **methionine**, and how the relationship

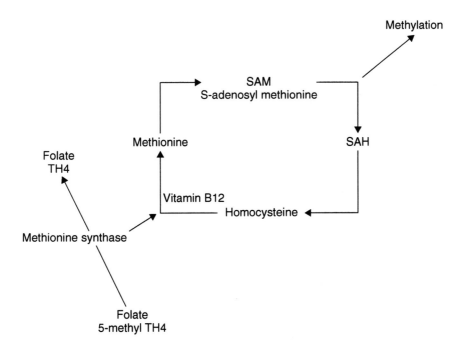

Figure 9.1 Homocysteine pathway.

between these two amino acids might also impact on, or be impacted by, the availability of something we've talked about before, **folic acid**. It's a complicated and incomplete picture but one of the suggestions is that high levels of homocysteine present in cases of autism might reflect issues with the regeneration of methionine from homocysteine.

If you'll remember back to our earlier discussions on genetics and epigenetics, one of the key epigenetic mechanisms is the **methylation** of **DNA** – adding something called a methyl group affecting the activity of genes – which is a process linked to methionine and a derivative called S-adenosyl methionine (SAM). For any interested reader, there is quite a bit of literature out there about this whole process and how, alongside elevated levels of homocysteine, DNA methylation levels may be perturbed in cases of autism.[302]

Just in case we've not confused you enough, we also made mention earlier in this book of a gene called ***MTHFR*** which controls production of a great Scrabble word for you, methylenetetrahydrofolate reductase (*MTHFR*). *MTHFR* is an **enzyme** which basically provides the body with the active form of folic acid needed to complete all that homocysteine to methionine palaver. With autism (and quite a few other conditions) in mind, there has been a suggestion of issues with the *MTHFR* gene controlling the amount of enzyme produced.[303] Indeed such issues may very well fit into those claims about supplementing folic acid and potentially reducing the risk of offspring autism.[20]

Stopping

We've tried to strike a balance throughout this book to provide you with some information about the science of autism with a specific focus on diet and food, but at the same time not overload you with the very weighty biochemistry. This chapter has been quite heavy going, but as you've probably already appreciated, autism is a complicated condition.

For those of you who do want a little more science about autism, we might recommend that you have a look at various areas showing some research promise, governing things like glutathione and its link to oxidative stress in autism[304] and the body of work looking at sulphate (sulfate) and autism[305] including some interesting discussions about another **mucolytic** agent called **NAC – N-acetyl cysteine**[306] with autism in mind. Who knows, if this book turns out to be a best seller, we might even write more about these issues.

References

265. Dohan FC. *et al.* Relapsed schizophrenics: more rapid improvement on a milk- and cereal-free diet. *Br J Psychiatry*. 1969; 115: 595–596.
266. Okusaga O. *et al.* Elevated gliadin antibody levels in individuals with schizophrenia. *World J Biol Psychiatry*. 2013 Jan 3.
267. Severance EG. *et al.* Complement C1q formation of immune complexes with milk caseins and wheat glutens in schizophrenia. *Neurobiol Dis*. 2012; 48: 447–453.
268. Niebuhr DW. *et al.* Association between bovine casein antibody and new onset schizophrenia among US military personnel. *Schizophr Res*. 2011; 128: 51–55.
269. Severance EG. *et al.* Gastrointestinal inflammation and associated immune activation in schizophrenia. *Schizophr Res*. 2012; 138: 48–53.
270. Severance EG. *et al.* Anti-gluten immune response following *Toxoplasma gondii* infection in mice. *PLoS One*. 2012; 7: e50991.

271. McCann D. *et al.* Food additives and hyperactive behaviour in 3-year-old and 8/9-year-old children in the community: a randomised, double-blinded, placebo-controlled trial. *Lancet.* 2007; 370: 1560–1567.

272. Kanarek RB. Artificial food dyes and attention deficit hyperactivity disorder. *Nutr Rev.* 2011; 69: 385–391.

273. Pelsser LM. *et al.* Effects of a restricted elimination diet on the behaviour of children with attention-deficit hyperactivity disorder (INCA study): a randomized controlled trial. *Lancet.* 2011; 377: 494–503.

274. Pelsser LM. *et al.* A randomised controlled trial into the effects of food on ADHD. *Eur Child Adolesc Psychiatry.* 2009; 18: 12–19.

275. Evangeliou A. *et al.* Application of a ketogenic diet in children with autistic behavior: pilot study. *J Child Neurol.* 2003; 18: 113–118.

276. Herbert MR. & Buckley JA. Autism and dietary therapy. *J Child Neurol.* May 2013.

277. Ruskin DN. *et al.* Ketogenic diet improves core symptoms of autism in BTBR mice. *PLoS ONE.* 2013; 8: e65021.

278. Neal EG. *et al.* The ketogenic diet for the treatment of childhood epilepsy: a randomised controlled trial. *Lancet Neurol.* 2008; 7: 500–506.

279. Konstantynowicz J. *et al.* A potential pathogenic role of oxalate in autism. *Eur J Paediatr Neurol.* 2012; 16: 485–491.

280. Brown AS. *et al.* Elevated maternal C-reactive protein and autism in a national birth cohort. *Mol Psychiatry.* 2013. doi: 10.1038/mp.2012.197.

281. Zerbo O. *et al.* Is maternal influenza or fever during pregnancy associated with autism or developmental delays? Results from the CHARGE (CHildhood Autism Risks from Genetics and Environment) study. *J Autism Dev Disord.* 2013; 43: 25–33.

282. Beumer W. *et al.* The immune theory of psychiatric diseases: a key role for activated microglia and circulating monocytes. *J Leukoc Biol.* 2012; 92: 959–975.

283. Morgan JT. *et al.* Microglial activation and increased microglial density observed in the dorsolateral prefrontal cortex in autism. *Biol Psychiatry.* 2010; 68: 368–376.

284. Hughes V. Microglia: the constant gardeners. *Nature.* 2012; 485: 570–572.

285. Heuer L. *et al.* Association of a *MET* genetic variant with autism-associated maternal autoantibodies to fetal brain proteins and cytokine expression. *Transl Psychiatry.* 2011; 1: e48.

286. Nordahl CW. *et al.* Maternal autoantibodies are associated with abnormal brain enlargement in a subgroup of children with autism spectrum disorder. *Brain Behav Immun.* 2013; 30: 61–65.

287. Braunschweig D. *et al.* Maternal autism-associated IgG antibodies delay development and produce anxiety in a mouse gestational transfer model. *J Neuroimmunol.* 2012; 252: 56–65.

288. Money J. *et al.* Autism and autoimmune disease: a family study. *J Autism Child Schizophr.* 1971; 1: 146–160.

289. Mouridsen SE. *et al.* Autoimmune diseases in parents of children with infantile autism: a case-control study. *Dev Med Child Neurol.* 2007; 49: 429–432.

290. Kakleas K. *et al.* The prevalence and risk factors for coeliac disease among children and adolescents with type 1 diabetes mellitus. *Diabetes Res Clin Pract.* 2010; 90: 202–208.

291. Ashwood P. & Van de Water J. Is autism an autoimmune disease? *Autoimmun Rev.* 2004; 3: 557–562.

292. Al-Ayadhi LY. & Mostafa GA. Elevated serum levels of interleukin-17A in children with autism. *J Neuroinflammation.* 2012; 9: 158.

293. Okada H. *et al.* The 'hygiene hypothesis' for autoimmune and allergic diseases: an update. *Clin Exp Immunol.* 2010; 160: 1–9.

294. Velasquez-Manoff M. *An Immune Disorder at the Root of Autism.* The New York Times. 2012. http://www.nytimes.com/2012/08/26/opinion/sunday/immune-disorders-and-autism. html (accessed July 2013).

295. Baieli S. *et al.* Autism and phenylketonuria. *J Autism Dev Disord.* 2003; 33: 201–204.

296. Tani Y. *et al.* Decrease in 6R-5,6,7,8-tetrahydrobiopterin content in cerebrospinal fluid of autistic patients. *Neurosci Lett.* 1994; 181: 169–172.

297. Frye RE. *et al.* Tetrahydrobiopterin as a novel therapeutic intervention for autism. *Neurotherapeutics.* 2010; 7: 241–249.

298. Novarino G. *et al.* Mutations in BCKD-kinase lead to a potentially treatable form of autism with epilepsy. *Science.* 2012; 338: 394–397.

299. Filipek PA. *et al.* Relative carnitine deficiency in autism. *J Autism Dev Disord.* 2004; 34: 615–623.

300. Celestino-Soper PB. *et al.* A common X-linked inborn error of carnitine biosynthesis may be a risk factor for nondysmorphic autism. *Proc Natl Acad Sci USA.* 2012; 109: 7974–7981.

301. Kałużna-Czaplińska J. *et al.* A focus on homocysteine in autism. *Acta Biochim Pol.* 2013 Jun 6.

302. James SJ. *et al.* Metabolic biomarkers of increased oxidative stress and impaired methylation capacity in children with autism. *Am J Clin Nutr.* 2004; 80: 1611–1617.

303. Pu D. *et al.* Association between *MTHFR* gene polymorphisms and the risk of autism spectrum disorders: a meta-analysis. *Autism Res.* 7 May 2013. doi: 10.1002/aur.1300.

304. Main PA. *et al.* The potential role of the antioxidant and detoxification properties of glutathione in autism spectrum disorders: a systematic review and meta-analysis. *Nutr Metab (Lond).* 2012; 9: 35.

305. Alberti A. *et al.* Sulphation deficit in 'low-functioning' autistic children: a pilot study. *Biol Psychiatry.* 1999; 46: 420–424.

306. Hardan AY. *et al.* A randomized controlled pilot trial of oral N-acetylcysteine in children with autism. *Biol Psychiatry.* 2012; 71: 956–961.

In conclusion

If you've reached this part of this book, congratulations and thanks for reading but don't go just yet as we have some parting words for you. Hopefully we've provided a comprehensive yet readable overview of autism, its complexity and variability, and of how dietary intervention might fit in with at least some cases of autism. Hopefully too those recipes and very practical hints and tips around feeding habits and times are going to be helpful for those thinking a GFCF diet might be for them.

We know you probably don't need reminding but we're going to say it anyway, **nothing included in this book is intended as medical or related clinical advice**. That and the fact that whilst we have perhaps come across as enthusiastic for the evidence and ways that dietary intervention might be working in cases of autism, we're not necessarily advocating that the GFCF diet is right for everyone nor that it is a cure-all for every negative aspect of autism or any of its comorbidities. People are complicated and any intervention put forward for autism or its comorbidities should not assume anything else.

It is perhaps customary to finish our journey with some profound phrase or saying which encapsulates this book. We were particularly drawn to a quote by novelist Jules Verne: 'Science, my lad, is made up of mistakes, but they are mistakes which it is useful to make, because they lead little by little to the truth.' Never a truer word has been spoken about the science of autism research. Many thanks for reading.

About the authors

Mark is a chef by trade and a successful entrepreneur who is involved in several enterprises and business investments. Mark was the founder of the award-winning Food Education Company in which he sold his interest in 2012. Mark has coupled his business knowledge with his catering and education experience to develop and launch innovative and creative businesses. Mark believes passionately in the importance of health, wellbeing and education combined with igniting a passion and belief in young people that they too can succeed in life. Mark's businesses represent his success in these fields and reflect his passion for developing innovative businesses and creating healthier communities. In addition to running businesses Mark also provides healthy food demonstrations with a difference, where he entertains and inspires audiences for clients in a wide range of sectors together with campaigns and media work. In 2011 Mark was asked to join the Percy Hedley College board of governors, which he immediately jumped at, having been involved with the foundation for seven years. Being involved with Percy Hedley has provided Mark with first-hand experience of the challenges faced by parents and professionals who care for individuals with autism.

Elouise is a dietitian who studied at Leeds Metropolitan University. During her placement year she found a passion for working around health prevention. Invited back by the public health team she spent time with to work with them after completing her degree, allowed Elouise the opportunity to work with families, education settings food companies and catering departments. Moving on Elouise then specialised in working around health promotion for children, including working to support families with all types of food allergies and conditions and who require therapeutic diets out in the community, to be able to have school meals. Elouise has a passion for cookery and developing new recipes and has written many recipes to support families including a recipe booklet for fussy eaters.

Paul is a researcher in autism and fairly well known (or at least he likes to think so) for his investigations into the use of dietary intervention for autism spectrum conditions. With a university educational background built up in the North East of England and based in psychology, he's spent over 15 years of his subsequent postgraduate research career examining various aspects of autism and has authored over 20 peer-reviewed papers on the topic including the results of experimental trials of the gluten- and casein-free diet for children with autism. He has a passion for science and the accurate communication of science forged during his doctoral studies and nurtured by various teaching duties and conference presentations. This led him to set up a blog about various facets of autism research as well as writing for several lay and professional journals and magazines on various science-related topics. The importance of food and diet to mental health and wellbeing represents the centre-point to his career, along with how the relationship between food and our physiology goes so much further than mere subsistence and physical health.

Glossary of terms

Please note that whilst we've reviewed all the terms included in this glossary, not everyone might agree with our descriptions.

ABA	Applied behavioural analysis is a learning approach used for autism whereby learning is broken down into simple steps and reinforced.
ADHD	Denotes attention deficit hyperactivity disorder, a developmental condition variably manifesting symptoms of inattentiveness and hyperactivity / impulsiveness
ADOS	The Autism Diagnostic Observation Schedule is an observational scheme which scores behaviour on set tasks to assess for the presence of autistic behaviours
A. muciniphila	*Akkermansia muciniphila* is a mucin-degrading bacterium found in the digestive tract
allergy	The chemical processes of the body reacting to something known as an allergen such as a food or other part of the environment
amino acid	Various important organic chemicals which combine to form peptides and proteins
antibiotic	Any medicine or compound which is able to inhibit the growth of or kill bacteria
antibody	A chemical produced by the immune system following the detection of a harmful substance called an antigen
ASCA	Anti-*Saccharomyces cerevisiae* antibodies reflect part of the current testing protocol to discriminate between the bowel conditions Crohn's disease and ulcerative colitis
ASD	Denotes autism spectrum disorder referring to a spectrum of developmental conditions variably manifesting autistic traits or features
Asperger syndrome	Part of the autism spectrum where language development is not usually affected
autoimmunity	A state whereby the immune system cannot differentiate between 'self' and foreign invaders such as bacteria or viruses and so mistakenly attacks healthy tissues
BAP	The broader autism phenotype refers to the subclinical presentation (not enough to merit a diagnosis of autism) of some of the features of autism

BH4	A naturally occurring compound which aids various enzymes concerned with the processing of certain types of amino acid
blood–brain barrier	The partly chemical–partly physical barrier which prevents chemicals or other materials in the blood entering the brain
branched-chain amino acids	A group of essential amino acids which the body cannot manufacture by itself (including valine, leucine and isoleucine)
Bristol Stool Chart	A medical chart used to categorise the various stool (poo) formations produced by humans
calcium	The most abundant mineral in the body, most of which is found in bone and teeth and supports their structure
carbohydrates	Chemical compounds normally associated with food and diet which release glucose, an important energy source for the body
carnitine	A compound derived from an amino acid which plays a role in energy production in the body
casein	The primary protein found in mammalian dairy sources such as milk, cheese and yoghurt
CDD	Childhood disintegrative disorder (CDD) or Heller's syndrome is a rare regressive developmental condition where, following a period of typical development, there is a marked loss of developmental and cognitive skills
CFS / ME	Chronic fatigue syndrome / myalgic encephalomyelitis are conditions characterised by chronic, debilitating and persistent fatigue post physical exertion
cholesterol	A fatty substance known as a lipid which is vital for various biological functions although in excess has been associated with various health and lifestyle complaints
C. difficile	Clostridium difficile is a type of bacteria that under certain circumstances can affect the digestive system and health and wellbeing
coeliac disease	An autoimmune condition affecting the digestive system caused by the ingestion of foods containing gluten
cofactor	A chemical which aids enzymes in their metabolising duties
comorbidity	The presence of one or more conditions in addition to a primary condition
cortisol	A steroid hormone which is released in response to stress
cytokine	Messenger chemicals secreted by cells of the immune system involved in processes such as inflammation
diabetes	Conditions which cause high blood sugar levels
DNA	Deoxyribonucleic acid encodes the genetic instruction manual
DSM	The Diagnostic and Statistical Manual is used to classify mental health and related problems
duodenum	The first part of the small intestine where the process of digestion continues
dysbiosis	A state of microbial (bacterial) imbalance normally associated with alterations in the levels of certain bacteria living in the digestive tract
EEG	Electroencephalography is a technique that records the electrical activity of the brain and is normally used to diagnosis epilepsy

endorphins	Naturally occurring chemicals which mimic some of the action of opioid – pain relieving – chemicals such as morphine
enzymes	Various essential chemicals which convert chemicals to other products in the body
epigenetics	Heritable and acquired modifications in the function of genes not due to changes to the DNA sequence
epilepsy	A set of neurological conditions affecting the brain that are primarily characterised by seizures
ESSENCE	Early symptomatic syndromes eliciting neurodevelopmental clinical examinations reflects the broader presentation of developmental and behavioural symptoms noted in various neurodevelopmental syndromes such as autism
ferritin	A protein found in cells which binds to iron and is used as an iron store
Feingold diet	An elimination diet which aims to remove from the diet sources of various artificial colours and preservatives that are suggested to impact on behaviour
fMRI	Functional magnetic resonance imaging is a technique looking at blood flow in the brain as a marker of brain activity
FMT	Faecal microbiota transplantation or a stool transplant involves transplanting a stool and its bacterial contents from a healthy donor to the digestive system of another person
folic acid	Vitamin B9 is important for the healthy development of the unborn baby including potentially modifying the risk of a child developing autism. It also helps convert carbohydrates into glucose.
FPIES	Food protein-induced enterocolitis syndrome is an unusual type of non IgE-mediated food allergy
fragile X syndrome	A genetic condition which causes a range of developmental problems including autistic-like behaviours
GABA	Gamma-aminobutyric acid is a neurotransmitter with a primarily inhibitory (calming) action
GAPS diet	The gut and psychology syndrome diet involves the removal of certain foods and the use of various fermented foods to support gut bacteria
GFCF diet	The gluten- and casein-free diet reflects a diet free from foods which contain the proteins gluten (from various cereal produce) and casein (from mammalian milk sources)
glutamate	An amino acid and powerful neurotransmitter affecting brain function
gluten	A storage protein found in various cereal grains such as wheat, barley and rye
GORD	Gastro-oesophageal reflux disease (GORD) also known as GERD is a digestive disorder characterised by heartburn and difficulty swallowing as a result of stomach acid rising into the oesophagus
gut	The gastrointestinal (GI) or digestive tract

gut–brain axis	The suggestion that gut and brain functions are interlinked and have the ability to influence each other
Guthrie test	The neonatal heel prick test used to collect a blood sample for testing for inborn errors of metabolism
HERVs	Human endogenous retroviruses are part of our genetic material and represent the remnants of our evolutionary exposure to viral infections
heterogeneity	Diversity in character, consistency or content. Its opposite is homogeneity, i.e. similarity in those aspects
homocysteine	An amino acid with potentially important health-related effects
IAG	Indolyl-acryloylglycine is a chemical derivative of the amino acid tryptophan
IBD	Inflammatory bowel disease refers to one of a number of conditions which affect various parts of the gut and are characterised by inflammatory changes
ICD	The International Classification of Diseases is used to classify disease and other health problems including those affecting mental health
ID	Intellectual disability also called learning disability refers to the presence of some intellectual or cognitive deficit normally linked to IQ
IgE	The immunoglobulin classically related to the process of allergy
ileum	The final part of the small intestine and the major site of vitamin B12 absorption
immunoglobulin	Chemicals made by the body and used by the immune system during the process of allergy or when the immune system identifies something foreign to the body
inflammation	The first response of the immune system following infection or injury characterised by pain, heat and swelling
iron	An essential mineral with various important functions in the body which when deficient can lead to a form of anaemia
jejunum	The middle section of the small intestine
ketogenic diet	A high fat, low carbohydrate diet which eventually puts the body into a state of ketosis as a result of using fat as an energy source rather than glucose (sugar) from carbohydrates
lactose	One of the main carbohydrates (sugars) found in mammalian dairy products normally metabolised by the lactase enzyme
leaky gut	Also called gut or intestinal hyperpermeability, leaky gut refers to a state whereby the gut membrane separating our digestive tract from the wider functions of the body is unusually porous
metabolic syndrome	A medical term which combines various biological measures (high blood pressure, diabetes, obesity) placing an individual at greater risk of certain lifestyle-related diseases
metabolomics	The study of the chemical fingerprint left behind by cellular processes in the body
methionine	An amino acid involved in the process of methylation, and important part of epigenetics, via its metabolite S-adenosyl methionine (SAM)

methylation	The addition of a chemical (methyl group) to parts of the genome subsequently affecting gene function
microbiomics	The study of the microbiome or the collected bacteria resident on or in the human body
microglia	A type of immune cell resident in the brain and spinal cord which looks for infections and damaged neurons
mineral	Compounds found in foods which the body uses for various important biological processes
mitochondria	The powerhouses of the cell involved in the conversion of food to energy which the body can use
MMA	Methylmalonic acid is produced when proteins break down, levels of which are linked to vitamin B12 deficiency
mRNA	Information in DNA is copied to messenger RNA via transcription. This information is translated to assemble a protein
MS	Mass spectrometry is a very precise analytical method used for the analysis of various chemicals in biological fluids
MTHFR	Methylenetetrahydrofolate reductase is an enzyme involved in the metabolism of folate (folic acid or vitamin B9)
mucolytic	Any chemical or bacteria or medicine which acts on mucus making it less thick and sticky
NAC	N-acetyl cysteine is a mucolytic and antioxidant chemical
non-coeliac gluten intolerance	A condition characterised by sensitivity to gluten but not showing the classical serological or genetic markers of more well-defined gluten-related conditions
OCD	Obsessive-compulsive disorder is a mental health condition characterised by obsessive thoughts and compulsive behaviours
oesophagus	Also known as the gullet, the oesophagus is the pipe through which food passes from the mouth to the stomach
opioid	A psychoactive chemical (acting on brain function and psychology) which binds to opioid receptors in the body involved in altering the sensation of pain
optimal outcome	A group of children defined by Fein and colleagues who having previously been diagnosed with an ASD were subsequently reported to show abatement of autistic traits to the point of no longer fulfilling the requirement for a diagnosis
OT	Occupational therapy refers to the assessment and treatment of various conditions to promote daily life skills and independent living
oxalate	A naturally occurring compound found in various plants and a primary constituent of kidney stones
PANDAS / PANS	Paediatric autoimmune neuropsychiatric disorders associated with streptococcal infections and Paediatric acute-onset neuropsychiatric syndrome are characterised by acute onset of the symptoms of obsessive-compulsive disorder (OCD) following an infection
parasite	An organism which lives in another organism (host) and derives nutrition from the host
peptide	Short chains of amino acids

phenotype	Observed behaviour or physiology as a function of the interaction of genetics and environment
pica	The consumption of non–edible objects or materials
PKU	Phenylketonuria is a genetic condition called an inborn error of metabolism which affects the metabolism of the amino acid phenylalanine and which, if left untreated, causes damage to the brain
PLP	Pyridoxal 5' phosphate is the active form of vitamin B6 which the body is able to use for various tasks
probiotic	A live bacteria suggested to confer some health benefit
propionic acid	A short chain fatty acid made by certain gut bacteria
RDoC	The Research Domain Criteria project by the US National Institute of Mental Health aims to classify psychopathology using dimensions of observed behaviour combined with various neurobiological measures
S. boulardii	*Saccharomyces boulardii* is a tropical strain of yeast which has been classified as a probiotic and is used to treat certain types of digestive disorder
ScanBrit	A randomised-controlled study of the gluten- and casein-free (GFCF) dietary intervention for autism
SCD	A specific carbohydrate diet limits the consumption of carbohydrates and restricts intake of refined sugars
schizophrenia	A mental health condition which affects the way a person perceives reality
serotonin	Also known as 5-HT, serotonin is a chemical involved in mood which originates from the amino acid tryptophan
social affect	A category combining issues with communication and social interaction used to describe autism
stomach	An important part of the digestive tract which contains acid and enzymes to help digest our food
Sutterella	A species of bacteria found in the digestive tract of people and animals
Th17	T helper 17 cells are specific cells of the immune system thought to play a key role in autoimmune conditions
tight junctions	The junctions between cells including those of the gut barrier
ToM	Theory of Mind is the process of understanding the intentions and feelings of others
tryptophan	A type of amino acid which is used to create the chemical neurotransmitter serotonin and the hormone melatonin
tTG	Tissue transglutaminase is an enzyme linked to the perpetuation of coeliac disease
vagus nerve	A nerve which travels from the brain stem down the body and is tasked with controlling various organs including the functions of the digestive tract
vitamin	Essential nutrients required for healthy functioning of the body
vitamin B6	A water-soluble vitamin which can exist in various forms and is involved in various biological reactions

vitamin B12	A water soluble vitamin which can exist in various forms, a deficiency of which can lead to a form of anaemia
vitamin D	A fat soluble vitamin which aids in the absorption of calcium as well as having various other important hormone-like functions in the body
zonulin	A protein that regulates the permeability of the intestines

Index